In Clinical Practice

Taking a practical approach to clinical medicine, this series of smaller reference books is designed for the trainee physician, primary care physician, nurse practitioner and other general medical professionals to understand each topic covered. The coverage is comprehensive but concise and is designed to act as a primary reference tool for subjects across the field of medicine.

Krsna Mahbubani

History Taking in Clinical Practice

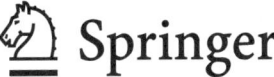
Springer

Krsna Mahbubani
West Hampstead Medical Centre
London, UK

ISSN 2199-6652 ISSN 2199-6660 (electronic)
In Clinical Practice
ISBN 978-3-031-29896-7 ISBN 978-3-031-29897-4 (eBook)
https://doi.org/10.1007/978-3-031-29897-4

© The Editor(s) (if applicable) and The Author(s), under exclusive license to Springer Nature Switzerland AG 2023
This work is subject to copyright. All rights are solely and exclusively licensed by the Publisher, whether the whole or part of the material is concerned, specifically the rights of translation, reprinting, reuse of illustrations, recitation, broadcasting, reproduction on microfilms or in any other physical way, and transmission or information storage and retrieval, electronic adaptation, computer software, or by similar or dissimilar methodology now known or hereafter developed.
The use of general descriptive names, registered names, trademarks, service marks, etc. in this publication does not imply, even in the absence of a specific statement, that such names are exempt from the relevant protective laws and regulations and therefore free for general use.
The publisher, the authors, and the editors are safe to assume that the advice and information in this book are believed to be true and accurate at the date of publication. Neither the publisher nor the authors or the editors give a warranty, expressed or implied, with respect to the material contained herein or for any errors or omissions that may have been made. The publisher remains neutral with regard to jurisdictional claims in published maps and institutional affiliations.

This Springer imprint is published by the registered company Springer Nature Switzerland AG
The registered company address is: Gewerbestrasse 11, 6330 Cham, Switzerland

Foreword

I always found history taking the trickiest skill to learn in medical school. Yet, it is the most important skill you will learn as a clinician.

As a medical student and even during my GP training, I found that learning history taking by grouping it into symptoms was very effective. When I became a clinical tutor, I taught my students using this technique and the feedback received was excellent. This was where the idea for this book came from. I want this book to be your guide as you learn about the different physiological systems and specialities.

When you take a history, you want to exclude anything urgent or any condition that can harm the patient quickly. Once you exclude this, then you need to think about other common conditions which could present with that symptom. The questions you ask in the history need to actively confirm or refute these diagnoses. There are tables interspersed within this book where I will ask you to write down key differential diagnoses for each of the common presenting complaints. Use this as your guide when thinking about scenarios and how to approach them.

The aim of this book is not to teach you everything about each and every clinical condition, and you will need to read around these conditions. However, I want you to familiarise yourself with what kinds of conditions you need to think about when presented with a symptom. The best way to know if you've understood everything is to practice, practice, practice. I have put in some patient examples to discuss, as well as some example OSCE stations at the back of the book. Before we start, I think it is important to revisit the basics of history taking.

Dr Krsna Mahbubani
West Hampstead Medical Centre,
London, UK

Contents

1. **Basic History Taking** 1
   - Presenting Complaint 1
   - History of Presenting Complaint 1
   - Past Medical History 2
   - Drug History 2
   - Family History 2
   - Social History 2
   - Systems Review 3
   - Taking a Pain History 4
2. **Cardiorespiratory** 7
   - Chest Pain 7
     - Cardiovascular Causes 7
     - Respiratory Causes 8
     - Gastrointestinal Causes 9
     - Muskuloskeletal 10
   - Shortness of Breath 13
     - Acute Causes 14
     - Chronic Causes 15
   - Palpitations 17
   - Cough 19
3. **Abdominal** 21
   - Abdominal Pain 21
     - Right Upper Quadrant (RUQ) 21
     - Epigastric 23
     - Left Upper Quadrant (LUQ) 24
     - Right/Left Loin 24
     - Right/ Left Iliac Fossa (RIF/LIF) 25

Contents

Suprapubic	26
Umbilical	26
Diarrhoea and Vomiting	26
Diarrhoea and Vomiting together	26
Vomiting Only	27
Diarrhoea Only	28
Constipation	30
Lower Urinary Tract Symptoms (LUTS)	32
Incontinence	33
4 Neurological	35
Headache	35
Recurrent/Chronic Headaches	37
Visual Changes	39
Dizziness/Vertigo	44
Collapse	46
Confusion	49
Numbness and Tingling	52
Peripheral Neuropathy	53
Mononeuropathy	53
Multiple Sclerosis (MS)	55
Anxiety	55
Peripheral Vascular Disease	56
Weakness	56
Acute Weakness	56
Sub-Acute/Chronic Weakness	56
Distal Weakness	58
Proximal Weakness	58
Motor Neurone Disease	58
Myasthenia Gravis	59
Tremor	60
5 Musculoskeletal	63
Joint Pains	63
Inflammatory Vs Mechanical Joint Pains	63
Rheumatological Causes	63
Orthopaedic Causes	64
Monoarthritis	65
Back Pain	65
Mechanical/Orthopaedic	66

	Rheumatological	67
	Infective	67
	Malignant	67
6	**Other**	**69**
	Leg Swelling	69
	Bilateral Leg Swelling	69
	Unilateral Leg Swelling	70
	Lumps and Bumps	71
	Cardio/Respiratory	72
	Neurological Histories	73
	Abdominal Histories	74
	Rheum/Ortho Histories	75
	Cases to Practice	76
7	**Gynaecology**	**93**
	Abnormalities of the Menstrual Cycle	93
	Menorrhagia	93
	Gynaecological Causes	93
	Systemic Causes	94
	Dysmenorrhea	94
	Gynaecological Causes	95
	Amenorrhea	95
	Primary Amenorrhea	95
	Secondary Amenorrhea	97
	Abnormal Bleeding Patterns	99
	Intermenstrual Bleeding	99
	Post-Coital Bleeding	100
	Post-Menopausal Bleeding	100
	Abnormal Pain	101
	Dyspareunia	101
	Superficial Dyspareunia	101
	Deep Dyspareunia	101
	Pelvic Pain	101
	Acute Pelvic Pain (Table 7.2)	102
	Chronic Pelvic Pain (Table 7.3)	102
	Example Answers	104
	Obstetrics and Gynaecology	105
	Gynaecological History	105
	Obstetric History	106
	Obstetric Nomenclature	106

8 Obstetrics ... 107
Abnormal Bleeding during Pregnancy ... 107
Abnormal Pain during Pregnancy ... 108
Itching in Pregnancy ... 109
   Dermatological Causes ... 109
   Systemic Causes ... 110
Vomiting in Pregnancy ... 110
Practice Cases ... 112

9 Paediatric Histories ... 119
The Febrile Child ... 119
Respiratory tract ... 119
   Common Viral Respiratory Tract
   Infections in Children ... 119
   Bacterial Respiratory Tract Infections
   in Children (Table 9.2) ... 120
Urinary Tract Infections ... 121
Gastrointestinal ... 121
Other Viral Infections (Table 9.3) ... 122
Rarer Causes of Fever in a Child (Table 9.4) ... 122
Enuresis—Bed Wetting ... 124
Abdominal Pain ... 125
   Acute Abdominal Pain ... 125
   Chronic Abdominal Pain ... 127
Failure to Thrive ... 128
Developmental Disorders ... 129
   Motor Delay ... 129
   Speech and Language Delay ... 130
Rashes in Children ... 131
   Acute Rashes (Table 9.8) ... 131
   Chronic Rashes ... 131
The Limping Child ... 133
   With Fever ... 133
   Without Fever ... 134
      Questions to Ask in a Child with a Limp ... 134
Paediatric Cases to Practise ... 136

10 Psychiatry ... 143
Low Mood ... 143
Anxiety/Worry ... 145
Hallucinations ... 146
Cases to Practise ... 148

Chapter 1
Basic History Taking

Presenting Complaint

This is a one line summary of what the patient has come in with e.g. chest pain, shortness of breath, palpitations.

History of Presenting Complaint

This is the most important part of the history. The questions should be specific to the presenting complaint. It is important to exclude all the life-threatening differentials. For example, if someone presents with shortness of breath, it is essential to rule out myocardial infarction or pulmonary embolism. It is also important to ask any red flags and to enquire about whether the patient needs immediate treatment or not.

Red Flags

These are symptoms which would suggest a more sinister pathology e.g. cancer.

Depending on the presenting complaint, these may be necessary to ask about and we will discuss them throughout the book.

Past Medical History

Here you should ask about any medical conditions the patient has.
You should ask about:

1. Current or previous medical conditions
2. Any surgeries
3. If you are taking a gynaecology history you should ask about the obstetric history of the patient i.e. have they had children and mode of delivery
4. In paediatrics, it may be relevant to ask about the delivery of the child/baby and how many weeks the child was when they were born—premature children are more prone to getting complications with certain diseases.

Drug History

Ask about

1. Any allergies to medications
2. Current medications they take, the dose and what time of day it is taken
3. It may be useful to enquire about any medications recently stopped
4. It is also important ask about any medications they are taking over the counter, as some patients may not volunteer this information.

Family History

Ask about any diseases which run in the family.

Social History

Enquire about smoking, drinking and any recreational drug use.

If relevant you should ask about how many pack years someone has smoked.

1 pack year = smoking 20 cigarettes a day for 1 year.

Therefore, if someone smokes 10 a day for 20 years that is $10/20 \times 20 = 10$ pack years.

$$\text{no. of cigarettes a day} / 20 * \text{number of years smoked} = \text{number of pack years}$$

In an older patient, you should ask about their housing situation. Where do they live, who they live with, if they have stairs, what their mobility is like i.e. can they walk unaided or do they need a frame. You can ask about if they have any carers at home and if they are independent of their activities of daily living (ADLs). These include washing and dressing themselves.

The social history in an older patient is important to get a picture of what their living conditions are like. Accordingly, this will help us decide if they will need occupational therapy or social services to establish a package of care.

ICE—Ideas, Concerns and Expectations

It is always important to ask the patient what they think is going on? This may give you an insight into any anxieties they may have.

Systems Review

At the end of your history, it is important to ask general questions to make sure you have not missed anything. I like to run down from head to toe and ask about:

headaches
visual problems
chest pain
shortness of breath

abdominal pain
changes to bowel/ bladder
back or joint pains

Taking a Pain History

Pain is an extremely common symptom that patients present with.

A common mnemonic which is used to assess pain is SOCRATES.

- **S**—site of the pain i.e. where is it?
- **O**—onset of the pain—did it come on suddenly or gradually?
- **C**—character of the pain. A lot of conditions have very characteristic types of pain which I have documented in the table below.
- **R**—radiation - does it radiate anywhere else?
- **A**—Associated symptoms such as vomiting
- **T**—time course – does it come and go? How long does it last?
- **E**—exacerbating/ relieving factors—what makes it better or worse?
- **S**—severity - > how severe is the pain. You can ask them to rate the pain using a scale of 0-10 where 0 is no pain and 10 is the worst pain they can ever imagine.

Examples of different pain 'characters' (Table 1.1).

This table is merely a general summary. In practice, there are many more pointers which will help you make a diagnosis.

I am now going to go through common presenting complaints and conditions which may present with each of them.

TABLE 1.1 This table shows the common types of pain you will encounter in history taking and causes of these

Type of pain	Site	Character	Radiation	Exacerbating factors
Cardiac chest pain	Left side of chest	Pressure 'Like someone sitting on you'	Jaw and left arm	Exertion can often make it worse
Gastritis	Epigastric	Burning pain	Sometimes extends up the chest in the distribution of the oesophagus	Spicy foods, alcohol
Respiratory/pleuritic	Anywhere in the chest	Usually respiratory problems present with sharp pains		Breathing in, coughing
Gastro-intestinal pain e.g. colitis, biliary colic	Anywhere in the abdomen	Cramping, aching	Depends on the cause	Again depends on the cause. For example if the cause is gallstones, then fatty foods often make it worse.

Chapter 2
Cardiorespiratory

Chest Pain

This is an exam classic and a very common presenting complaint.

Let's start by breaking it down.

What system malfunctions can chest pain be a symptom of. I can think of four (Table 2.1):

Cardiovascular Causes

- Reduced oxygen supply to the heart can cause angina or in the worst case a myocardial infarction. Angina/MI presents as *crushing* left sided chest pain. The pain can radiate to the jaw and left arm. It is classically described as a pressure sensation or 'elephant sitting on your chest'. Additionally, the patient may also present with shortness of breath or dizziness.
  - In stable angina the chest pain will usually come on after walking a fixed distance.
  - In unstable angina or a myocardial infarction, the pain may be at rest or on walking a shorter distance.

TABLE 2.1 This table demonstrates the causes of chest pain you may encounter in clinical practice. They are divided into different systems

Cardiovascular	Respiratory	Gastrointestinal	MSK
*Myocardial infarction (MI)	*Pulmonary embolism (PE)	*GERD	*Costochondritis
*Angina	*Pneumonia		
*Arrhythmias	*Pneumothorax		
*Aortic dissection			
*Pericarditis			

The umbrella term for any condition causing a reduction in blood supply to the heart is 'ischaemic heart disease' or IHD for short.

Risk factors of IHD include diabetes, smoking, hypertension and high cholesterol. Palpitations may accompany a cardiac cause of chest pain as well.

- Pericarditis is a term for inflammation of the outer lining of the heart. The pain is a *sharp* pain that is worse on lying down and is alleviated by sitting forward. Causes of pericarditis include infection, cancer, autoimmune disease.
- Dissection is a condition which results in a tear within the internal lining of an artery (Fig. 2.1). If this occurs in the aorta, the pain is a *sharp tearing pain* that radiates through to the back or neck. As with the other cardiac causes of chest pain, they may also have dizziness and shortness of breath.

Respiratory Causes

- Any respiratory cause of chest pain tends to be *pleuritic* (sharp and worse on breathing in).
- Cough, fever and sputum may help identify a pneumonia. The cough is often productive of green or yellow phlegm.

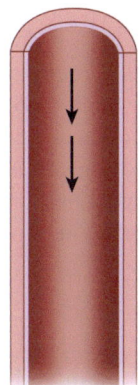 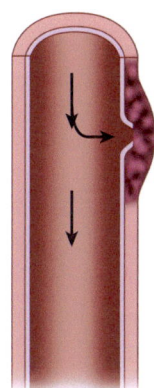

Figure. 2.1 This diagram shows a tear in the lining of the artery resulting in dissection. This accumulation of blood in the artery lining will reduce the amount of blood being delivered to the target organs. It can also result in rupture of the artery

- A pulmonary embolism (PE) is a clot in the vasculature of the lung. If someone has a PE, they will likely also be short of breath. They may also have leg swelling (DVT). Risk factors for a PE include taking the contraceptive pill, smoking, underlying cancer, immobility, high blood pressure and high cholesterol.

Gastrointestinal Causes

- Reflux presents as a *burning* pain. This can affect the epigastric area as well as the central chest.
- Symptoms worse on eating, as well as any associated belching/ burping may indicate reflux. Specific triggers include spicy foods, alcohol, stress. Sometimes the acid coming up can leave a metallic taste in the mouth and can also trigger coughing.

Muskuloskeletal

- Costochondritis is muscle inflammation in the chest. It is a *sharp* pain, worse on breathing in and also worse on movement. The key to identifying costochondritis is that the pain is worse when touching the inflamed area.
- Costochondritis may be triggered by trauma or injury to the chest. The pain is typically worse on movement or pressure.

Here is an exercise you can do to help understand the causes of chest pain. Fill in the table with the causes of chest pain that are important to rule out when faced with a history.

P.S. You can recreate this table for any presenting complaint and is a good way to ensure you have understood a topic.

Cause	Type of pain	Associated symptoms	Risk factors

Example answers (Table 2.2).

TABLE 2.2 This table shows the symptoms of common causes of chest pain

Cause	Type of pain	Associated symptoms	Risk factors
Myocardial infarction	Pressure like pain on the left side of the chest	Shortness of breath, dizziness, palpitations	High blood pressure, high cholesterol, smoking, diabetes
Pericarditis	Sharp pain across the chest—worse on lying down	Shortness of breath, dizziness	History of cancer, autoimmune or recent infection.
Dissection	Tearing pain going from chest to the neck and to the back	Shortness of breath, dizziness	High blood pressure, high cholesterol, aortic aneursym
Pulmonary embolus	Sharp chest pain worse on breathing in	Shortness of breath	Deep vein thrombosis, high blood pressure, smoking, diabetes
Reflux	Burning epigastric pain and central chest pain	Burping, belching, nausea	Consumption of spicy foods, caffeine or alcohol, having a hiatus hernia

Jeremy

I was a GP trainee in my first ever GP job when I came across Jeremy. He walked into my room and sat down very comfortably. He was in his late 40's and had an unremarkable medical history. He had barely been to the doctors in the last few years.

I started my consultation by asking, as I always do, how I could help him that day.

He replied by saying that he had developed some chest pain over the last few days which was unusual for him. On further questioning, the pain was sharp and pleuritic, and he also had shortness of breath. He had no risk factors for a pulmonary embolism and no symptoms of a DVT.

His examination was incredibly unremarkable and I was a little unsure what could be causing his symptoms. Although he described breathlessness, his saturations were 96%.

I was torn what to do. One of the differentials which I was still unable to rule out was a pulmonary embolism. I discussed my concerns with him and he agreed to go to hospital for blood tests and a chest X-ray.

A few weeks later I received a discharge summary from the hospital. Jeremy had been diagnosed with multiple pulmonary embolisms secondary to a lung cancer.

The learning from this case is to trust your gut and to try and identify the red flags in the history. Pleuritic chest pain and shortness of breath in the absence of infective symptoms could be a pneumothorax or pulmonary embolism which needs further work up.

> **Chris**
>
> I was doing a routine clinic at a GP surgery. My next patient was a 25 year old man, Chris. He had developed some left sided shoulder pain which was radiating all the way to his right. He was also experiencing some shortness of breath and felt something wasn't quite right. The pain came and went, and he found lying down on his right side very difficult. He had experienced something similar a year ago and was told it was musculoskeletal pain. He did not have a fever and was otherwise fit and well. His examination findings were unremarkable, however during the consultation he felt quite dizzy and nauseous. His heart rate was fluctuating slightly. Although initially I thought this could be muscular given his age, I decided to send him into hospital given how unwell he was feeling. He was later diagnosed with pericarditis.
>
> This was an interesting case as had no risk factors for pericarditis. It is important to keep this in mind in anyone presenting with new onset sharp chest pain.

Shortness of Breath

There is a lot of overlap between a chest pain and shortness of breath history, as the causes are very similar.

Let's brainstorm causes of shortness of breath by system (Table 2.3). With a shortness of breath history it is also important to ask exactly how long the symptom has been going on for.

The next step is to think of other associated symptoms that can help put the pieces together.

TABLE 2.3 This table demonstrates the causes of shortness of breath you may encounter in clinical practice. They are divided into different systems and into how quickly the symptoms may develop

	Cardiovascular	**Respiratory**	**Other**
Acute	*MI *Unstable angina *Arrhythmia	*Pneumonia *Pneumothorax *Pulmonary embolism *Asthma/COPD exacerbation	
Chronic	*Heart failure *Valve disease	*COPD *Asthma *Interstitial lung disease *Malignancy	*Anaemia

Acute Causes

Any chest pain? (see above). Cardiovascular causes may present with chest pain, shortness of breath and palpitations as we discussed above.

- Pneumothorax and PE's are usually sudden onset and present with sharp chest pain along with shortness of breath.
- The risk factors of a PE were discussed above.
- A pneumothorax is a collapsed lung. It also presents with pleuritic chest pain and shortness of breath. It can occur after trauma; Therefore it is important to inquire about any physical trauma if you suspect a pneumothorax. A pneumothorax can also occur without trauma. A spontaneous pneumothorax (in the absence of trauma) can be primary or secondary.
    - A primary pneumothorax is one which occurs in a lung with no underlying lung disease. It is often linked to a certain phenotype—tall, thin male.
    - A secondary pneumothorax can occur in people with underlying lung disease e.g. COPD.

Chronic Causes

- Heart failure is the term given to a condition in which the heart is unable to pump blood efficiently. Heart failure typically presents with shortness of breath on exertion due to fluid build-up in the lungs. There is also shortness of breath when lying flat (orthopnoea). Other symptoms which may also be present include swelling of the legs and/or abdomen. Causes of heart failure include ischaemic heart disease and previous MI's (this damages the wall of the heart). Heart valve diseases also result in heart failure symptoms as they reduce the outflow of blood from the heart.
- Interstitial lung disease (ILD) is a disease that results in fibrosis of the lung tissue, which in turn reduces optimal gas exchange. It has an insidious onset and presents with shortness of breath on exertion. Patients may also complain of a dry cough, weight loss and lethargy. ILD is typically idiopathic i.e. we do not know what the underlying cause is. However other causes include:
    - Drugs—use of methotrexate or long term nitrofurantoin use can trigger ILD
    - Environmental triggers: long term exposure to irritants such as asbestos and mould can cause hypersensitivity pneumonitis.
    - Chemotherapy can also trigger ILD
- Malignancy (lung cancer) may present with **red flags** such as weight loss, night sweats, loss of appetite and a cough. Patients may notice that they cough up blood (haemoptysis). This is an important red flag in respiratory histories. Lung cancer is often, but not always, linked to smoking. Exposure to other toxic substances such as asbestos can also increase risk of lung cancer.
- Asthma and chronic obstructive respiratory disease (COPD) are both respiratory conditions which cause a narrowing of the airways resulting in shortness of breath. Asthma occurs due to reversible inflammation in the airways. Asthma is linked to atopy and allergy, and onset is usually in childhood

or early adulthood. Symptoms may be triggered by an allergen (e.g. dust, pollen, viral infection) of some sort. It is important to ask about pets, medications and occupation. Chronic asthma symptoms are usually worse in the morning or late at night. Classic symptoms are wheeze, breathlessness and cough. There may also be chest tightness. In any asthma history, you should ask about previous hospital admissions for nebulisers or any intensive care admissions, as this will help you gauge how sick they can get.
- COPD is secondary to lung damage due to smoking and onset is often later in life. Similar to asthma, it presents with shortness of breath and wheeze. It is a progressive disease and unlike asthma the airway narrowing is not reversible. Over time, patients develop a reduced exercise tolerance and many suffer from shortness of breath at rest. It is important to ask about smoking in all respiratory histories. This includes other drugs too, such as cannabis.

Mary

Mary was an elderly lady who came into my clinic room feeling incredibly short of breath. She had no chest pain, however the shortness of breath was slowly worsening to the extent that she could only walk a few metres before feeling breathless. She had a fairly unremarkable past medical history—only some long standing acid reflux for which she took over the counter gaviscon. On further questioning she had no other significant symptoms: no orthopnea, no leg swelling.

Her chest was clear, however she did have a very loud systolic murmur. My initial thought was that she may have a valve lesion such as aortic stenosis. I sent her off for blood tests and an echo. Her blood results came back a few days later with an Hb of 68. She had not had any blood tests in a while and it was unclear how long she had been anaemic for. I referred her to hospital where she had a transfusion. An endoscopy was

> performed which showed a bleeding ulcer and she was treated with high dose omeprazole.
>
> This case was a useful reminder that shortness of breath is not only caused by cardiac or respiratory causes. Severe anaemia can also cause breathlessness in patients.

Palpitations

The word palpitations has been mentioned a few times already. Palpitations are irregular heart rhythms which can manifest as a fast heart beat.

There are many causes of palpitations. Some arrhythmias result in the patient having a cardiac arrest. The main cause of this is ventricular fibrillation which will not be discussed here. Other causes of tachycardias include:

- Atrial fibrillation—this is a condition which causes an IRREGULARLY IRREGULAR heart beat. It is diagnosed with an ECG that must have both an irregular heart rhythm and the absence of p waves.
- Supraventricular tachycardia—the arrhythmia is triggered by an abnormal pathway above the ventricles. On an ECG the QRS complex is narrow (smaller than 3 small squares).
- Ventricular tachycardia—the arrhythmia is triggered by abnormal pathways at the level of the ventricles. On an ECG the QRS complex is broad (larger than three small squares).
- Sinus tachycardia—this is a fast heart beat in the absence of any conduction abnormality. Patients may have this secondary to drugs (salbutamol can trigger a tachycardia), fever, dehydration, anxiety.

Alongside an abnormally fast heart beat, patients may also experience chest pain and dizziness or a collapse with loss of consciousness. This is because the irregular rhythm makes it much harder for the heart to maintain an adequate cardiac output.

Atrial fibrillation causes an irregular heart rhythm whereas the other tachyarrhythmias are regular.

The causes of tachyarrhythmias can be grouped as follows (Table 2.4):

When taking a palpitation history it is important to ask the following:

- When did the palpitations start/ how long has the patient been experiencing them?
- How long do they last for?
- Are they regular or irregular? If they describe an irregular heartbeat it is likely that this is atrial fibrillation.
- Do they experience any chest pain, shortness of breath or dizziness? This will tell you if there is any haemodynamic instability
- Try to determine any cause e.g. ask about symptoms of hyperthyroidism

TABLE 2.4 This table demonstrates the various causes of arrhythmias

Electrolyte disturbances	Electrolyte abnormalities such as hypo/hyperkalaemia and hypo/hypercalcaemia can cause rhythm disturbances
Genetic	Conditions such as long QT syndrome and wolf parkinson white syndrome can predispose someone to arrhythmias. These can be diagnosed on an ECG
Structural	Structural abnormalities in the heart such as cardiomyopathies can make someone more predisposed to arrhythmias
Ischaemic heart disease	Following an MI, the structural damage can increase the risk of arrhythmias
Infections	Sepsis can trigger arrhythmias
Stimulant/drug induced	Stimulants such as caffeine and drugs such as cocaine may trigger arrhythmias
Endocrinological	Thyrotoxicosis can predispose an individual to tachyarrhythmias such as atrial fibrillation

Cough

The next symptom we are going to tackle is cough.

The causes of a cough can also be broken down into systems (Table 2.5).

- A Chest infection presents with fever, productive cough and sometimes breathlessness.
- Lung cancer presents with a chronic cough. There may also present with red flags such as weight loss, loss of appetite and haemoptysis (coughing up blood). Risk factors for developing lung cancer include smoking, cannabis use and also asbestos exposure.
- The cough in asthma is classically described to occur at night or early morning. There may be specific triggers and associated wheeze. These patients may have other symptoms of atopy such as eczema and food allergies. (See previous section on shortness of breath).
- Bronchiectasis is a condition caused by chronic lung damage, commonly as a result of previous chest infections and childhood infections. The bronchioles become thickened and enlarged resulting in frequent infections. Patients may also have some haemoptysis at times.
- COPD is a combination of bronchitis and emphysema. It causes a chronic cough, shortness of breath on exertion as well as wheeze.

TABLE 2.5 This table demonstrates the causes of cough you may encounter in clinical practice. They are divided into the different systems

	Respiratory	**Cardiovascular**	**Gastrointestinal**	**Other**
Acute	*Pneumonia/ viral respiratory tract infection			
Chronic	*Lung cancer *COPD *Asthma *Bronchiectasis	Heart failure	Reflux	*Drugs *Post nasal drip

- Heart failure (see shortness of breath chapter)
- Reflux can present with a burning pain behind the sternum. It is often triggered by spicy foods or alcohol. Don't forget to ask for risk factors which may suggest a bleeding ulcer—vomiting (more specifically vomiting blood), or any change in bowel habit or blood in the stool.
- Ace inhibitors typically cause a dry cough in some patients. The cough is a common reason why some patients are unable to tolerate these medications.
- Post nasal drip occurs due to mucus dripping down from the nose to the back of the throat. This causes some irritation resulting in a cough. It is common in patients with rhinitis or following a viral respiratory infection.

Chapter 3
Abdominal

Abdominal Pain

Abdominal pain is slightly more complex as its cause depends on where the pain in the abdomen is.

You can use the diagram below as a rough guide (Table 3.1). Think of the organs present in each part of the abdomen (go back to your anatomy textbook and correlate the diseases to the organs).

As the list of causes is too large to group together, let's tackle it area by area.

Right Upper Quadrant (RUQ)

This is usually related to liver or gall bladder (Figure 3.1). Common diseases which present with pain in this region are:

- Biliary colic—this is due to gallstones. It presents with an ache after eating a fatty meal.
- Cholecystitis—this is an infection of the gallbladder often due to an impacted stone in the cystic duct. It presents with constant pain in the RUQ and fever. On examination, the patient will be **Murphy's sign** positive. Murphy's sign is when the patient develops severe pain during inspiration whilst a doctor presses over the gallbladder.

TABLE 3.1 This table describes the causes of abdominal pain based on the location of pain. Usually this correlates to the anatomy of the abdomen

Right upper quadrant Hepatitis Biliary colic Cholecystitis Lower lobe pneumonia	**Epigastric** Peptic ulcer disease Pancreatitis Atypical chest pain (commonly seen in posterior myocardial infarction)	**Left upper quadrant** Splenic pathology Lower lobe pneumonia
Right loin Pyelonephritis Polycystic kidney disease Renal colic Other renal disease	**Umbilical** Gastroenteritis IBS Coeliac disease Bowel obstruction Ischaemic bowel Aortic aneurysm Diabetic ketoacidosis	**Left loin** Pyelonephritis Polycystic kidney disease Renal colic Other renal disease
Right iliac fossa Ovarian cyst Ectopic pregnancy Appendicitis Terminal ileitis	**Suprapubic** Period pain Fibroids Cystitis Pregnancy symptoms miscarriage	**Left iliac fossa** Ovarian cyst Ectopic pregnancy Diverticular disease Diverticulitis

- Ascending cholangitis—this occurs due to an infected, blocked common bile duct. It presents with a triad of fever, jaundice and rigors. It can quickly cause the patient to become septic so must be treated quickly.
- Conditions which affect the liver can also cause pain in the right upper quadrant.

    *Hepatitis is an acute infection or inflammation of the liver. It can be caused by viruses (Hepatitis A, B and C) and rarely can be secondary to autoimmune disease. Liver disease can also cause jaundice and an increased tendency to bleed (the liver is important in the production of clotting factors).

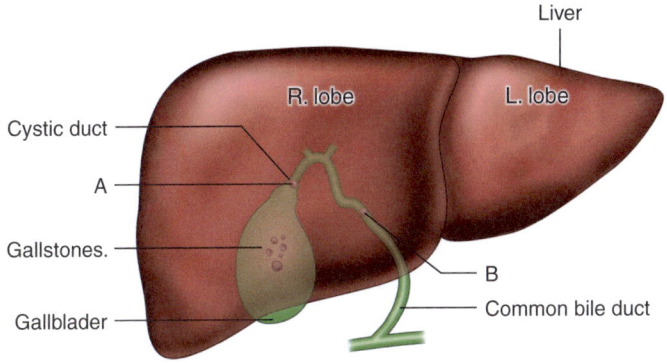

Figure 3.1 This image shows the anatomy of the biliary tract. Point A shows where a stone may be impacted to cause cholecystitis and point B shows where the stone may be impacted resulting in ascending cholangitis

> *Chronic damage to the liver as a result of alcohol, fatty liver, cancer and autoimmune conditions can cause cirrhosis. Cirrhosis does not always cause abdominal pain, but patients will have ascites, prominent veins visible in the abdomen, jaundice and easy bruising.

Epigastric

- The stomach and the pancreas are both located in the epigastric region.
- Burning epigastric pain is typical of gastritis. Patients may complain that the burning pain is extending up the chest into the throat. It is usually triggered by hot, acidic or spicy foods as well as alcohol. If the gastritis leads to an ulcer this can bleed causing hematemesis (blood in the vomit) and malena (stool with old blood in it—which often looks black and sticky or tar like)

- Pancreatitis causes epigastric pain radiating to the back. The patient will also be vomiting. Causes of pancreatitis can be remembered with the mnemonic—GET SMASHED

    G—gallstones
    E—ethanol
    T—trauma
    S—steroids
    M—mumps
    A—autoimmune disease
    S—scorpion sting
    H—hypercalcaemia
    E—ERCP
    D—drugs

Left Upper Quadrant (LUQ)

This is rarely a presenting complaint so we will not focus on this. The spleen is the main organ in the left upper quadrant.

Right/Left Loin

The loins are where the kidneys are located. The two main causes of loin pain are

1. Pyelonephritis—In its simplest form this is infection of the kidney. It usually starts off as a urinary tract infection with suprapubic pain and dysuria. However, if the infection ascends to the kidney, it can lead to loin pain, fever and in severe cases sepsis.
2. Renal colic—this classically presents as loin to groin pain. It is extremely painful. Patients may also have haematuria. The management depends on the size of the stone. Small stones (<5 mm) may pass themselves, however larger stones will need some sort of intervention.

Right/ Left Iliac Fossa (RIF/LIF)

1. The iliac fossa is where the ovaries are kept. Therefore, any ovarian pathology will lead to pain in the left or right iliac fossa. This includes ovarian cysts, ectopic pregnancies and ovarian torsion.
2. Appendicitis—this is inflammation of the appendix. The appendix is found in the right lower quadrant of the bowel. It presents with central abdominal pain that migrates to the right iliac fossa. Patients may also be nauseous and lose their appetite. It is diagnosed with an ultrasound or CT scan and the management is usually removal of the appendix.
3. Diverticulitis—diverticula are outpouchings of the gut as a result of increased pressure (Figure 3.2). Therefore people who have suffered from constipation often suffer from rectal diverticula. They usually cause no problems, however if they become infected it can cause pain in the left lower quadrant, diarrhoea and sometimes PR bleeding. It is treated with antibiotics.

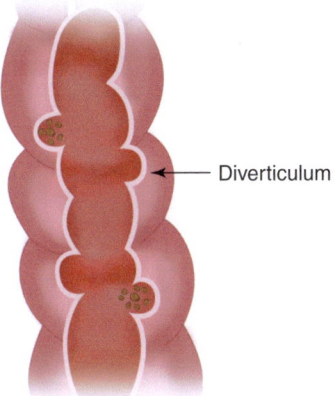

FIGURE 3.2 This diagram shows the outpouching in in the gut wall which is called a diverticulum

Suprapubic

1. The suprapubic area is where the bladder is located. Therefore cystitis (UTI) often presents with suprapubic pain. Other symptoms include pain on passing urine and going to the toilet more frequently.
2. As well as the bladder, in women the uterus is also located in the suprapubic region. Therefore, gynaecological causes can also lead to pain there. These include fibroids, period pains and pelvic inflammatory disease. Often these are accompanied by other symptoms including — vaginal bleeding (can be heavy and painful) and vaginal discharge. This is discussed more in the gynaecology chapter.

Umbilical

1. This part of the abdomen is often affected in gastroenteritis which causes generalised 'crampy' abdominal pain.
2. Bowel obstruction can also cause generalised abdominal pain. This is caused by a blockage in the bowel which obstructs the flow of food down it. There is more about this condition in the next section.
3. Coeliac disease and irritable bowel syndrome (IBS) can also cause some generalised pain. I will discuss this in more detail in the next section.

Diarrhoea and Vomiting

These symptoms can occur together or separately, and often the differentials are different.

Diarrhoea and Vomiting Together

Most often this is due to gastroenteritis. In a gastroenteritis history it is important to ascertain the fluid status of the patient. You should ask the following:

- How often are they vomiting?. The colour of vomit is also important to ascertain, and if there is any blood. Vomiting blood is a red flag which suggests a more serious pathology.
- Are they able to drink sips of fluid (if they cannot, then they may need IV fluids)
- Any abdominal pain or distention? How much diarrhoea are they passing and how often? Is there any blood in the stool?
- How much urine are they producing and what colour is it (reduced frequency of urine output is a sign of dehydration and might indicate that the patient needs IV fluids)
- You should also ask about any co-morbidities which may complicate the infection
- e.g. diabetes (being unwell with diabetes can increase sugar levels)
- In women you should ask about the chance of pregnancy.
- It is also important to ask about possible source of infection (eating out, any unwell contacts).

*Blood in the vomit or stool is a red flag and may suggest that this is not a simple gastroenteritis. One of the differentials for diarrhoea and vomiting is a bleeding ulcer. This can cause hematemesis (blood in the vomit) and melaena (black soft tarry stool which has a typical pungent smell).

Vomiting Only

Differentials for this include

1. Gastroenteritis (see above)
2. Pregnancy—it is always important to ask about pregnancy and the date of the last menstrual period in women.
3. Bowel obstruction—this is important to rule out in a patient with vomiting and no diarrhoea. It occurs due to a blockage in the bowel which prevents the stool from passing through. This causes a backflow of faecal matter.

It presents with vomiting, often green or feculent in colour. These patients are constipated and <u>do not</u> pass wind too. They often have a distended abdomen as well.

Bowel obstruction can be divided into small bowel obstruction and large bowel obstruction depending on which part of the intestine is affected (Table 3.2).

4. If there is any blood in the vomit (haematemesis) the cause may be a bleeding ulcer.
5. Pancreatitis (see previous section)
6. Other causes: other rare causes to think about are:

    - Diabetic ketoacidosis—can also present with vomiting, and abdominal pain
    - Addison's disease—extremely rare!
    - Brain tumour (increased cranial pressure)

Red Flags
- Abdominal distention
- Absolute constipation (think bowel obstruction)
- Haematemesis—bleeding ulcer, oesophageal varices (a sign of liver disease), malignancy, Mallory Weiss tear

Diarrhoea Only

Differentials for this depends on if this is acute (new onset) or subacute (ongoing for a few weeks):

1. ACUTE

    - Gastroenteritis
    - Inflammatory bowel disease (can be subacute as well)

Table 3.2 This shows the causes of small and large bowel obstruction

Causes of small bowel obstruction	Causes of large bowel obstruction
Hernia	Bowel malignancy
Adhesions from previous surgery	Volvulus

- Diverticulitis
- Bleeding ulcer (presents with melaena therefore you need to ask about colour, smell and any associated haematemesis or epigastric pain)
- Overflow diarrhoea from chronic constipation
- Ischaemic bowel (Rare)

2. SUBACUTE

- Thyrotoxicosis
- Inflammatory bowel disease
- Coeliac disease
- Irritable bowel syndrome
- Diverticular disease
- Chronic pancreatitis
- Bowel cancer—any change in bowel habit in an older patient should prompt you to think about bowel cancer.
- Inflammatory bowel disease is an autoimmune condition which causes inflammation of the bowels. It usually presents with abdominal pain and a change in bowel habit. There are two main types of inflammatory bowel disease.

    (A) Crohn's disease—Crohn's disease can cause inflammation at any point in the gut from the mouth to the anus. It presents with abdominal pain and diarrhoea. A common site of pain is the right iliac fossa—this is because the terminal ileum is a commonly affected site in Crohn's disease which is situated in the right lower abdomen.

    (B) Ulcerative colitis—unlike Crohn's disease, this only affects the large bowel. It presents with diarrhoea which can be bloody.

- Coeliac disease is an autoimmune condition which is caused by gluten intolerance. Any gluten containing food can cause symptoms such as abdominal pain, diarrhoea and constipation.

> **Regina** was a 25 year old female who presented with bloody diarrhoea. She had recently been abroad and therefore the initial diagnosis was gastroenteritis. Her stool culture came back negative, however her symptoms persisted. Following this, a feacal calprotectin test was sent off to check for inflammatory bowel disease. There was a problem with the sample and therefore the result was delayed. In the meantime, her symptoms were so bad that she ended up going to A + E. An urgent colonoscopy was performed which showed that she had bowel cancer even though she was very young. On further questioning it transpired that she had been treated with radiotherapy for Hodgkin's lymphoma as a child. The radiation had increased her risk of developing another cancer. Although this is rare, always consider malignancy in a young person with a previous history of cancer or radiation treatment.

Constipation

The causes of constipation can range from localised to systemic causes.

1. Most commonly, constipation is due to not having enough fibre or water in the diet. Patients may need to take laxatives to help them open their bowels regularly.
2. Irritable bowel syndrome (IBS) is a condition which causes chronic abdominal pain and alternating diarrhoea and constipation. Usually the patient's symptoms including pain and bloating improve when they open their bowels. There is no organic cause of the symptoms and usually it is triggered by stress and poor sleep patterns.
3. A sudden change in bowel habit in an older person (either constipation or diarrhoea) should make you think about the possibility of cancer. Ask about other red flags such as weight loss, loss of appetite and lethargy.

4. As mentioned earlier, absolute constipation is a red flag and may indicate bowel obstruction.
5. Coeliac disease can also lead to constipation.
6. Constipation may also be related to gynaecological pathology. For example, ovarian cysts and cancers can press on the bowel and cause constipation. Often ovarian cancer can present like IBS with constipation and bloating. In an older patient with IBS type symptoms, consider investigating ovarian cancer.
7. There are also systemic causes of constipation including hypothyroidism and hypercalcaemia.

Kevin

I was an FY2 doctor in A + E when I met Kevin. He was a 75 year old man who was otherwise well. He had a history of an enlarged prostate for which he had recently had surgery for. He was otherwise well and only took tamsulosin. He presented to A + E with pain in his stomach 1 hour after eating an apple pie. He described the pain as burning in nature and constant. He had never suffered from reflux beforehand. He was initially triaged to the urgent care GP who administered some lansoprazole. The GP also checked his urine given his prostate history. She noted that his urine had some glucose, however he was not a known diabetic. She referred him to A + E for some blood tests to check his blood glucose. When I examined Kevin, he still had pain in his epigastric region, however his observations were stable. I decided to do a venous blood gas on him as well as the blood tests. I suspected this was a case of severe reflux or a stomach ulcer. To my surprise, I saw that his lactate on his blood gas was 5. The normal value is less than 2. Due to this, I requested a CT scan to rule out any perforation. To our surprise, the scan showed that he had developed small bowel obstruction and an ischaemic bowel and he was immediately taken to theatre. This was secondary to

> post-operative adhesions. This case was a very important learning experience for me. The main take home message was that any unusual pain in an older person should be taken seriously. Kevin had never suffered from reflux previously and it would be unusual to suddenly develop this in later life.

Lower Urinary Tract Symptoms (LUTS)

The urinary tract is located in the abdomen and therefore it is important to focus a little bit more on LUTS symptoms. LUTS describes any difficulty in passing urine. This includes:

- pain on passing urine (dysuria)
- urinary frequency
- difficulty initiating urination (hesitancy)
- poor stream
- nocturia (going frequently in the night)

The following table looks at different causes of LUTS symptoms (Table 3.3).

In an OSCE, if someone is describing LUTs symptoms it is often in the context of an elderly male with an enlarged prostate. in this situation it is important to ask the following:

- Any fever, burning or smelly urine? — to exclude a UTI
- Any changes to medication?
- Any red flags which may suggest cancer? — haematuria, weight loss, appetite loss and back pain. The back pain could be suggestive of bony metastases as prostate cancer can spread to the bones.
- Any urinary retention? — One of the risks of having an enlarged prostate is the potential to go into urinary retention. This is the inability to pass urine. It causes severe abdominal pain due to the bladder distension and is treated with insertion of a catheter.

TABLE 3.3 This table shows the causes of LUTS symptoms

Infection	Physiological	Malignancy	Drug induced
Both urinary tract infections and sexually transmitted infections can cause LUTS	In men, it is normal to experience some LUTS symptoms as the prostate enlarges with age. This is called benign prostatic hyperplasia (BPH)	In men, prostate cancer can cause LUTS symptoms In women, ovarian cancer can also trigger abnormal urinary symptoms as the mass presses on the bladder.	Taking diuretics can cause urinary frequency Caffeine can also have a mild diuretic effect on the body

Incontinence

Incontinence is a relatively common presenting complaint, especially in women. We can divide the types of incontinence into:

- Stress incontinence
  Stress incontinence occurs due to a weak pelvic floor muscle. It causes urine to leak when there is raised abdominal pressure such as when a person coughs or laughs. It is common in women following a vaginal delivery during childbirth. It is managed with pelvic floor exercises and lifestyle advice. In more severe cases, women can be referred for surgery.
- Urge incontinence
  This is another name for bladder muscle instability or overactive bladder. This occurs due to bladder muscle spasms which results in a sudden urge to pee and a tendency to leak urine if you do not go to the toilet on time. Causes of urge incontinence include (note this is not a complete list)

- nerve damage (e.g. in MS)
- Irritation of the bladder wall as a result of an infection or bladder stones
- low oestrogen levels due to the menopause
- Diabetes

- Mixed incontinence
  This is when patients have symptoms of both stress and urge incontinence.
- Overflow incontinence
  This occurs when the bladder is unable to empty normally (urinary retention). The bladder fills up, resulting in the leakage of urine due to overflow. Causes can be divided into:

  - Obstruction of the urine outflow tract: anything which causes an obstruction to the outflow of urine can result in urinary retention and therefore overflow. This includes bladder stones, prostate enlargement, malignancy in the urinary tract.
  - Damage to the nerves which control bladder function. Urinary retention is a symptom of cauda equina and in a patient with back pain and urinary retention you need to organise an urgent MRI to rule out cauda equina.

Chapter 4
Neurological

Headache

Headache histories are another exam classic.

The differential of headache will vary depending on if the headache is acute or chronic.

Let's start with ***acute headaches*** (Table 4.1).

Let's break it down by discussing the associated symptoms/ presentations:

1. Subarachnoid haemorrhage—This classically presents with a 'thunderclap' headache. This is a sudden onset headache typically felt at the back of the head. It is classically described as if someone has 'been kicked in the back of the head'. Associated symptoms include vomiting and neck stiffness. Subarachnoid haemorrhage is a medical emergency.

    Subarachnoid haemorrhages are usually due to rupture of an aneurysm, and risk factors for aneurysm development include those that are similar to ischaemic heart disease—hypertension and smoking. These both disrupt the lining of blood vessels which can lead to an aneurysm. (Patients with polycystic kidney disease are also more likely to have a brain aneurysm and are therefore at a higher risk of a subarachnoid haemorrhage).

TABLE 4.1 This table shows acute causes of headaches you may come across in clinical practice

Neurovascular	Infection	Eye	Rheum	Others
Bleed/ subarachnoid haemorrhage	Meningitis/ Encephalitis (Many viral conditions such as the flu and Covid can present with a mild headache)	Acute glaucoma	Temporal arteritis	Hypertension

2. Meningitis—this is an infection of the lining of the brain (the meninges). It presents with fever, photophobia (light troubling the eyes) and neck stiffness. There are a few different bacteria that can cause meningitis, including *Neisseria Meningitidis*. This particular bacteria causes 'meningococcal septicaemia' leading to the classic non-blanching rash associated with meningitis. Meningitis needs to be treated promptly with IV antibiotics.
3. Encephalitis is an infection of the brain matter itself. It presents with fever and acute confusion. It is a medical emergency.
4. Glaucoma is a condition which results in increased pressure in the eye. There are two types of glaucoma—open angle glaucoma and closed-angle glaucoma. The latter can present acutely with a red, painful eye. Vision may be blurred and a patient may complain of seeing haloes in their visual fields.
5. Temporal arteritis is a vasculitis of the temporal artery. It causes a headache in the temporal region of the head where the temporal artery lies. Another classical symptom of temporal arteritis is 'jaw claudication' in which the patient experiences jaw pain whilst eating.

    Temporal arteritis is closely linked to polymyalgia rheumatica and patients may also experience symptoms such as lethargy, malaise, shoulder and hip pain.

    Temporal arteritis is an important diagnosis to make, as if untreated it can lead to visual loss in that eye. It is treated with high dose steroids.

6. Do not forget that malignant hypertension can also present with a headache. It is always important to check blood pressure in any patient who has a headache.

Recurrent/Chronic Headaches (Table 4.2)

> **Leah is a 45 year old lady who presented** with pain in her hips and shoulders. I suspected a diagnosis of polymyalgia rheumatica and asked her to get some blood tests done. A few days later, she presented to A + E with severe pain around her left eye and reduced vision. She was subsequently diagnosed with temporal arteritis. This was an important reminder to always ask about eye symptoms in anyone with a suspected diagnosis of polymyalgia rheuamtica.

1. Migraines are a type of headache that tend to be recurrent. They are quite debilitating and are usually a unilateral pulsating headache. There may be associated nausea and vomiting as well as photophobia. Often patients say that they need to lie down in a dark room when they have a migraine.

    Some patients experience migraines with aura. This is important to ask about. Types of aura's include:

    - visual e.g. seeing zigzag lines
    - Tactile e.g. pins and needles
    - olfactory e.g. funny smells

    (Migraine with aura is a contra-indication to taking the combined pill as there is a very slight increased risk of stroke).

TABLE 4.2 This table lists common causes of chronic headaches

Recurrent	Chronic
Migraine	Tension headache
Cluster type headache	Analgesia overuse headache
	Space occupying lesion

Migraines may be triggered by certain things. These include:

- alcohol
- cheese
- chocolate
- stress
- menstruation

When taking a migraine history, try and work out what the trigger is. If the patient is unsure, ask them to keep a headache diary for 2 weeks to try and find any patterns in the cause of the headaches.

2. Cluster headache – A cluster headache is a type of recurrent headache which comes in clusters lasting weeks to months followed by periods without any symptoms (hence the name). It presents with a severe unilateral headache and pain around the eye. Often there may be some lacrimation of the eye. They are extremely debilitating and can stop individuals from sleeping well. Typically in an exam question the patient wants to 'bang his head against the wall' due to the severity of the pain.
3. Tension-type headache – This is described as a tight band around the head, squeezing inwards. It is often due to underlying stress that the patient may be experiencing.
4. Analgesia overuse headache – This is a headache which develops from regular use of painkillers for another type of headache e.g. tension type headache. As the painkillers wear off, the pain comes back. The mainstay of treatment is withdrawal of the medication. The symptoms will initially worsen, however over time the headache will get better.
5. Space occupying lesion – A space occupying lesion such a brain tumour will usually present with a headache. The mass will increase the intracranial pressure and often the headache is worse on lying flat or first thing in the morning. It often wakes them up at night and they may have some visual symptoms. The patient may also vomit.

Red flags to ask about in a history of someone with chronic headaches include anything that suggests raised intracranial pressure. These include:

- waking up in the night with pain
- pain worse on lying flat or bending forwards (this accentuates the raised pressure)
- increased vomiting associated with the pain
- visual symptoms

There are other benign causes of raised intracranial pressure but in anyone with red flags, a malignancy must be ruled out.

Visual Changes

Eye symptoms may accompany neurological conditions or be secondary to an ophthalmological problem (Figure 4.1).

Common problems with the eyes include (Table 4.3):

- *Any eye condition which causes sudden onset blurring of vision or visual loss needs to be referred straight to the eye casualty.

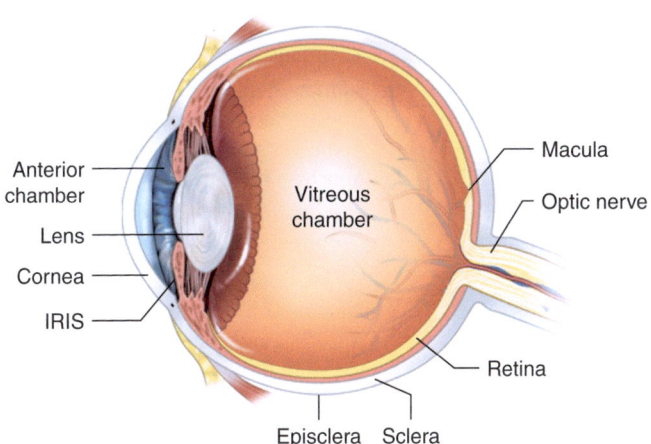

FIGURE 4.1 This diagram demonstrates the basic structure of the eye

TABLE 4.3 This table demonstrates the different visual symptoms you may encounter and the causes of these

Symptom	condition	Presentation
Red eye without pain	Conjunctivitis	This is a common infection of the eye resulting in redness and discharge of the eye. It can be caused by a bacterial or viral infection. There should not be any blurry vision and it is not very painful although there may be mild discomfort.
	Subconjunctival haemorrhage	This occurs due to burst blood vessels in the subconjuntival region. Causes of this include trauma or raised pressure (e.g. from coughing or sneezing). It can also occur if someone has high blood pressure. It is not painful and does not affect the vision.
Red eye with pain	Inflammatory eye condition e.g. scleritis, uveitis	This is inflammation of the sclera (outer part of the eye) or the uvea (the middle part of the eye). They can both cause pain, visual changes and photophobia. They are linked to autoimmune conditions such as inflammatory bowel disease and rheumatoid arthritis.
	Glaucoma	Acute glaucoma is caused by a sudden increase in eye pressure. Symptoms include a red, painful eye and associated headache. Patients may also have nausea and vomiting and have blurred vision. They also complain that they can see haloes.
	Corneal abrasion	This is damage to the cornea. It can be caused by trauma. The symptoms include a red, painful eye with associated blurred vision.
	Herpes simplex keratitis	This occurs when you get a herpes infection of the eye. Symptoms include a red eye, photophobia and blurred vision. The infection can cause a dendritic ulcer which can be seen when the eye is stained.

TABLE 4.3 (continued)

Symptom	condition	Presentation
Red eyelid	Stye	This presents as a lump on the eyelid. It is due to a buildup of debris in the oil glands. They do not affect vision and can take weeks to months to get better.
	Blepharitis	This is inflammation of the eyelid. It can lead to the eyelids feeling swollen and uncomfortable. It is associated with dry eyes and the patient may describe a gritty sensation in the eye.
	Periorbital cellulitis	This is an infection of the eyelid. The patient will complain of redness and swelling around the eye. They may also have a fever. It needs to be treated promptly as it can lead to orbital cellulitis which can damage the eye and cause reduced visual acuity.
Eye pain without redness	Optic neuritis	This is inflammation of the optic nerve which can cause reduced vision and painful eye movements. It is often one of the first symptoms of an underlying inflammatory condition such as MS.
	Dry eyes	Eyes will feel sore and gritty. It can occur as a result of environmental factors such as excessive screen use. In some cases there may be an underlying autoimmune disease (Sjogrens syndrome).

(continued)

TABLE 4.3 (continued)

Symptom	condition	Presentation
Acute visual loss	Amaurosis Fugax	This is loss of vision secondary to an embolus. It is described as a curtain coming down over the field of vision and is associated with transient ischaemic attacks.
	Retinal detachment	This is when the retina detaches from the back of the eye. Risk factors include having a previous retinal detachment, a family history of this or increasing age. It can cause permanent vision loss if untreated as the retina is detached from its blood supply. Symptoms include floaters in the visual field as well as flashes of light. Vision will be blurred and they may even complain of a dark shadow or curtain in their visual field.
	Vitreous detachment	The vitrea is a gel-like substance within the eye. It is connected to the retina, and as you get older it can start to pull away from the retina. This causes flashes and floaters in the visual field. Vitreous detachment can increase your risk of developing retinal detachment.

TABLE 4.3 (continued)

Symptom	condition	Presentation
Chronic visual loss	Cataracts	A cataract is a cloudy substance forming within the lens. They can occur with age and present with haziness of vision.
	Age related macular degeneration	The macula is a part of the eye which is important for central vision. Age related macular degeneration is a progressive disorder in which the macula is damaged. It results in a blurring and sometimes a complete loss of your central vision.
	Chronic glaucoma	Chronic open angle glaucoma can cause damage to the optic nerve secondary to the raised pressures. It usually causes a loss of peripheral vision first.
	Diabetic retinopathy	Uncontrolled blood sugars can damage the retina and the small blood vessels which supply it. This can lead to microhemorrhages and areas of ischaemia.
	Brain tumours	Certain brain tumours can cause damage to the optic tract which can affect visual fields. A classic example is a pituitary tumour which can compress the optic chiasm causing visual loss.

Dizziness/Vertigo

Dizziness can be divided into lightheadedness or vertigo.

Light-headedness describes a situation when someone is feeling faint or about to collapse. It is also known as pre-syncope. Causes of this include anything which can lower your blood pressure or cardiac output. There is an overlap between causes of light-headedness and collapse.

Causes include:

- Cardiac causes: heart failure, valve disease, arrhythmias, low heart rate (heart block). It is important to ask about cardiac symptoms such as chest pain, palpitations and shortness of breath.
- Other causes of low blood pressure:

    (a) postural hypotension
    (b) dehydration
    (c) sepsis

- Anaemia—This can cause dizziness as there is a reduced amount of oxygen being carried to the brain.

Vertigo on the other hand is a feeling that the room is spinning around you. It can cause nausea and vomiting due to the spinning sensation.

Causes of vertigo can be divided into the following (Table 4.4):

When taking a history of vertigo think about the acuteness of the symptoms.

*If the vertigo is <u>sudden onset,</u> think about vestibular neuritis, cerebellar stroke.
*If the history is <u>episodic,</u> the differential is likely to be BPPV, Merniers disease or migraine
*If the history is <u>chronic,</u> you need to exclude an acoustic neuroma or any other cause of cerebellar degeneration.

TABLE 4.4 This table demonstrates the causes of vertigo. They are divided into the different systems involved

Neurological	ENT	Other
Head injury—Concussion following head injury can cause vertigo	Labyrinthitis/vestibular neuritis—These are both caused by an infection of different parts of the inner ear. They cause sudden onset vertigo & nausea. Labyrinthitis may also cause hearing loss.	Drugs—Drugs such as gentamicin are ototoxic. Therefore, one of the side effects is damage to your hearing and balance.
Stroke—Brain stem and cerebellar stroke can lead to vertigo. Always consider this as a differential in an older patient with sudden onset vertigo.	Benign paroxysmal positional vertigo (BPPV)—This is a condition which is caused by a loose otilith in the inner ear apparatus. The patient develops vertigo in response to certain triggers. Often they will complain of vertigo when they turn their head.	
Acoustic neuroma—This is a type of brain tumour which originates from the eighth cranial nerve (vestibulocochlear nerve). It can cause the following symptoms due to compression of nearby structures: – Hearing loss – Changes to facial sensation – Loss of balance – Tinnitus	Meniere's disease is a condition which causes recurrent episodes of tinnitus, nausea, vertigo and a feeling of aural fullness. The exact cause of Merniere's is unknown but it can sometimes run in families.	

(continued)

TABLE 4.4 (continued)

Neurological	ENT	Other
Cerebellar disease—The cerebellum sits at the back of the brain. It helps control the coordination of movements. Damage to the cerebellum can cause vertigo and feeling off balance. Other symptoms and signs of cerebellar dysfunction include (DANISH): 　D—Dysdiadochokinesia 　A—Ataxia 　N—Nystagmus 　I—Intention tremor 　S—Slurred speech 　H—Hypotension		
Vestibular migraine—This is a type of migraine which presents with vertigo. There may also be nausea, headache and photophobia.		

Collapse

Collapse can lead to a temporary or prolonged loss of consciousness. Syncope is another word for a collapse. It is usually caused by insufficient blood flow to the brain. One of the commonest causes is a simple faint (vasovagal). In some circumstances, a collapse can be indicative of something much more sinister. This table describes some of the causes of a collapse (Table 4.5). There is some overlap between the causes of light-headedness and collapse as the former can lead to the latter.

When taking a collapse/ syncope history, it is a good idea to work out the series of events i.e. what happened before,

TABLE 4.5 This table gives examples of the different causes of collapse. They have been divided into the systems involved

Cardiac	Neurological	Reflex syncope	Orthostatic	endocrine
Arrhythmias	Epilepsy	Vasovagal	Postural drop in BP	Hypoglycaemia
Heart block	Stroke/bleed	Situational syncope e.g. micturition syncope		Addisons disease
Heart failure				
Valve abnormalities				

during and after the collapse. Always ask if there was a witness, as they might be able to give you more information.

- Cardiac causes of collapse are due to the inability of the heart to maintain perfusion to the brain. Both arrhythmias and heart failure can reduce cardiac output. Patients may have preceding symptoms such as chest pain or palpitations. It is also important to ask about any symptoms of heart failure.
- Vasovagal is another word for a simple faint. It occurs due to a drop in blood pressure in response to certain triggers. Common triggers include dehydration, the sight of blood, feeling very hot or an intense emotional experience. The person usually regains consciousness really quickly. They may have a few twitches (which could look like a seizure), however this is very brief and there is no post-ictal phase.
- Epilepsy leads to abnormal movements in the arms and legs. The patient would usually not be able to remember this, which is why a witness is important. During the seizure, they may bite their tongue or pass urine (urinary incontinence). After the event, the patient may be drowsy for 1–2 h (the post ictal phase).
- Of note, epilepsy is not the only cause of a seizure. Other causes of seizures include:

    1. space occupying lesions
    2. dementia
    3. electrolyte abnormalities
    4. hypoglycaemia
    5. withdrawal from drugs such as alcohol

- Hypoglycaemia is the term for low blood sugar. If the blood sugar drops below 4 mmol/l this can cause symptoms such as dizziness, tremors, confusion and eventually collapsing. It is important to check the blood sugar in any patient who has had a collapse.
- Addison's disease is a rare endocrinological condition in which an individual does not produce enough cortisol (stress hormone). The symptoms include weakness, fatigue and low blood pressure. It can lead to a person collapsing

if the cortisol levels are significantly low. This is termed 'Addisonian crisis'.
- Orthostatic blood pressure is when there is a large drop in blood pressure on standing up. Causes include dehydration, blood pressure medication or diuretics, neurological diagnoses such as Parkinson's disease and even Addison's disease.
- In some individuals, certain triggers can cause syncope. This is termed situational syncope. A common cause is micturition syncope when a person faints whilst passing urine. The cause of this is not completely understood but is likely to be related to stimulation of the vagus nerve resulting in a drop in blood pressure.

Confusion

Confusion can be described as a clouding of consciousness. Medically we can objectively identify confusion using the abbreviated mental test score or AMTS. Usually a score of 6 or less is suggestive that the patient is confused.

The following table shows the questions to ask in the abbreviated mental test (Table 4.6):

Confusion can be both acute or chronic. An acute confusional state is also known as delirium. Let's start by discussing acute confusion in a patient.

The causes of delerium include (Table 4.7):

If a patient has chronic confusion, this is termed dementia. There are various different types of dementia:

(a) Alzheimer's disease

Alzheimer's disease is a gradual deterioration in memory due to atrophy of the brain. It tends to start with a loss of short term memory loss and the key feature is a gradual and steady deterioration in memory.

(b) Vascular dementia

Vascular dementia can occur in patients who have had strokes. Often, but not always, there is a stepwise deterio-

TABLE 4.6 The questions in the abbreviated mental test score

What is your age?
What is the time (to the nearest hour)?
Where are you (e.g. name of hospital, clinic)?
Repeat an address (42 West Street). Ask them to recall this at the end
Recognise 2 people e.g. doctor and nurse
What year are we in?
Name the president/ prime minister/ monarch
What is your date of birth?
Dates of a historical event e.g. world wars
Count backwards from 20 to 1

ration in memory triggered by subsequent cerebrovascular events.

(c) Lewy Body dementia

Lewy body dementia can be thought of as a combination of dementia and Parkinsonism. Patients will develop bradycardia, rigidity and tremors. In addition, they will also have memory loss and suffer from frequent falls. Patients with Lewy Body dementia are also classically known to suffer from visual hallucinations—usually of people or animals.

(d) Frontotemporal dementia

Frontotemporal dementia is also known as Pick's disease. It is often caused by neuro-degeneration. This type of dementia can result in a personality change in the patient.

When taking a history from a patient with dementia it is very important to assess how safe they are. Questions you should ask include:

– Do they live in a flat or house
– Who lives with them
– Have they ever wandered out of the house and got lost

TABLE 4.7 This table shows the causes of delirium

Infection	Ischaemia	Electrolyte Disturbance	Drugs/alcohol	Medication
Intracranial infections such as meningitis and encephalitis Sepsis and severe infections of any kind. Other, more rare, causes include tropical infections such as malaria In older patients even milder infections such as a UTI can cause delirium.	Patients can develop confusion after a stroke	e.g. Hypo/hypernatramia Hypo/hypercalcaemia	Drug intoxication and withdrawal	*Sleeping tablets such as benzodiazepines *Opiates such as tramadol *Oral steroids can also cause confusion in patients.

- Have they ever left the gas on at home by mistake
- Any falls
- How they manage with their activities of daily living.

These questions are important to give us an idea about what type of care package the patient may need. If they have family with them, there may be no need for carers.

If they live alone, they may eventually need carers coming in to help with meals and medication. In severe cases, the patients are unable to look after themselves or are at risk of neglect or accidental harm. In these situations, a care home may be the most appropriate place for them to stay. These decisions need to be taken together with next of kin.

Another important aspect of managing a patient with dementia is mental capacity. The mental capacity act sets out important legislation on what decisions can be made on behalf of a person who lacks mental capacity. The first rule is always to assume a person has capacity regardless of the medical history. It is our duty as clinicians to ensure that we provide our patients with all the important information about any treatment that they may need. We then need to assess capacity by checking if they can:

1. Understand the information provided
2. Retain the information
3. Weigh up the pro's and con's
4. Communicate their decision

If a patient is deemed not to have capacity then we can act in their best interests. It is important to check if they have an advanced directive or have appointed a power of attorney.

Numbness and Tingling

Let's discuss causes (Table 4.8):

TABLE 4.8 Table showing the causes of altered sensation of the skin

Neurological	Psychological	Vascular
Peripheral neuropathy	Anxiety	Peripheral vascular disease
Mononeuropathies		
Multiple sclerosis		

Peripheral Neuropathy

This term is used to describe a condition in which there is damage to the nerves at the distal end of arms and/or legs (Figure 4.2).

It can be sensory, motor or both. Pins and needles are a sign of sensory involvement.

The numbness usually spreads proximally in a glove and stocking distribution.

Symptoms include numbness, tingling or abnormal sensations such as burning or stabbing pains.

There are many causes of sensory peripheral neuropathy including:

- Diabetes
- Chronic alcohol use
- B12 deficiency
- Cancer (neuropathy can be a paraneoplastic syndrome)
- Chronic kidney disease
- Autoimmune disease

Mononeuropathy

This describes damage to a single nerve.

The common ones you will come across are in the following table (Table 4.9). It can cause both sensory and motor symptoms.

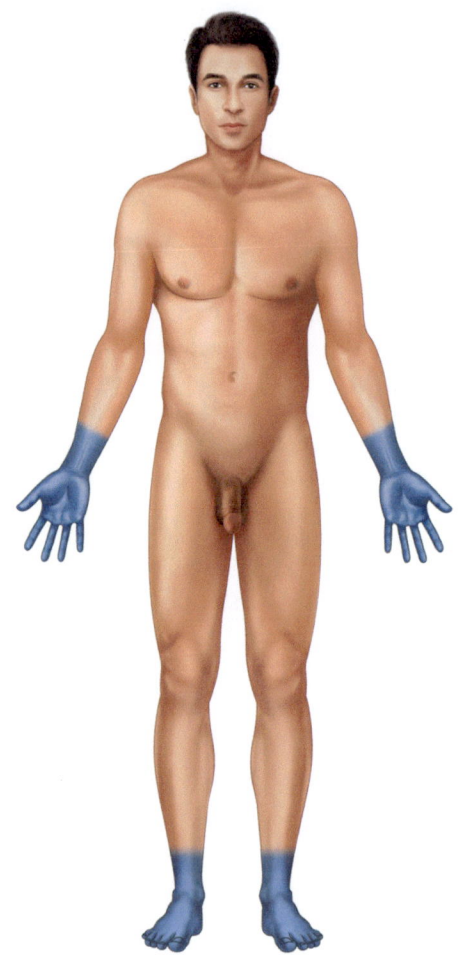

Figure 4.2 The following diagram shows where the sensory loss is in a patient with peripheral neuropathy. You can see why it is called the glove and stocking distribution

TABLE 4.9 This table shows common mononeuropathies

Syndrome	Symptoms
Carpal tunnel	This occurs when there is damage to the median nerve at the wrist. It causes pins and needles in the fingers, especially the thumb, index finger and middle finger.
Ulnar neuropathy	This occurs due to damage to the ulnar nerve. The specific symptoms depend on where the nerve is damaged. The sensory symptoms include numbness to the ring and little finger which are supplied by the ulnar nerve. Motor symptoms include a partial claw hand due to inability to straighten the ring and little finger.
Radial nerve damage	Damage to the radial nerve can cause numbness to the back of the thumb, index and middle finger. It also causes wrist drop as the radial nerve supplies the muscles which control extension of the wrist.
Common peroneal nerve damage	Damage to the common peroneal nerve causes foot drop.

Multiple Sclerosis (MS)

Multiple sclerosis is a condition which leads to demyelination of nerves in the brain and the spinal cord. It can affect different nerves at different times and can cause weakness and numbness of the arms and legs. The key piece of information in the history which is suggestive of MS is that the symptoms occur in different areas of the body at different times with periods of recovery in between.

Anxiety

Anxiety and panic attacks in patients can cause symptoms such as chest pain, palpitations and feeling on 'edge'. It is often accompanied by numbness and tingling due to hyperventilation. There may be triggers for this, however some patients can get panic attacks without any obvious triggers.

You can use a beta blocker such as propranolol to help treat the symptoms. Patients will also need psychological therapies such as CBT (cognitive behavioural therapy) as well as possibly antidepressant medications.

Peripheral Vascular Disease

Peripheral vascular disease is caused by a reduction in blood supply to the legs. A common symptom is pain in the legs when walking that improves with rest (intermittent claudication). Due to the lack of blood flow, patients can also experience numbness in the legs. On examination, the foot pulses may be weak or absent. The leg may be cold to touch. Red flag symptoms include pain at rest or at night, or change in colour of the leg to red blue or black.

Weakness

Weakness is the term used to describe reduced muscle strength in an individual. The weakness may be focal or generalised. The causes can be divided into acute and chronic (Table 4.10).

Acute Weakness

Sub-Acute/Chronic Weakness

This can be divided into different causes as follows (Figure 4.3):

Weakness 57

TABLE 4.10 This table shows common causes of acute weakness

cause	symptoms
Stroke	A stroke causes focal neurological weakness depending on where the stroke is. A stroke will cause contralateral symptoms to the side of the brain that is affected. Symptoms include weakness in the arms, legs and/ or slurred speech. As a stroke affects the upper motor neurones, the affected limbs will be stiff and spastic.
Multiple sclerosis	As discussed earlier this can cause episodes of acute weakness during periods of demyelination. The symptoms resolve between flares.
Guillain Barre syndrome	This is a condition which affects the distal nerves and causes a rapidly ascending paralysis. It is triggered by an infection such as gastroenteritis caused by *campylobacter*.
Botulism toxicity	*Botulinum* is an anaerobic bacteria which produces a toxin. Botulinum toxin blocks the production of the neurotransmitter acetylcholine thereby affecting muscle function. Often people get infected by eating tinned foods which have been contaminated.

Distal Weakness

1. CIDP stands for chronic inflammatory demyelinating polyneuropathy. It is a progressive demyelinating condition which affects motor and sensory function. It starts distally and progresses proximally. It can be thought of as a chronic version of Guillain Barre syndrome.
2. Hereditary motor and sensory neuropathies (HMSN) are a group of conditions which result in damage to the peripheral nerves. Charcot Marie Tooth disease is a type of HMSN. Symptoms include weakness and loss of sensation in the distal limbs. In the legs it can lead to foot drop. The muscle wasting can cause what appears to be an 'inverted champagne bottle' appearance of the feet.

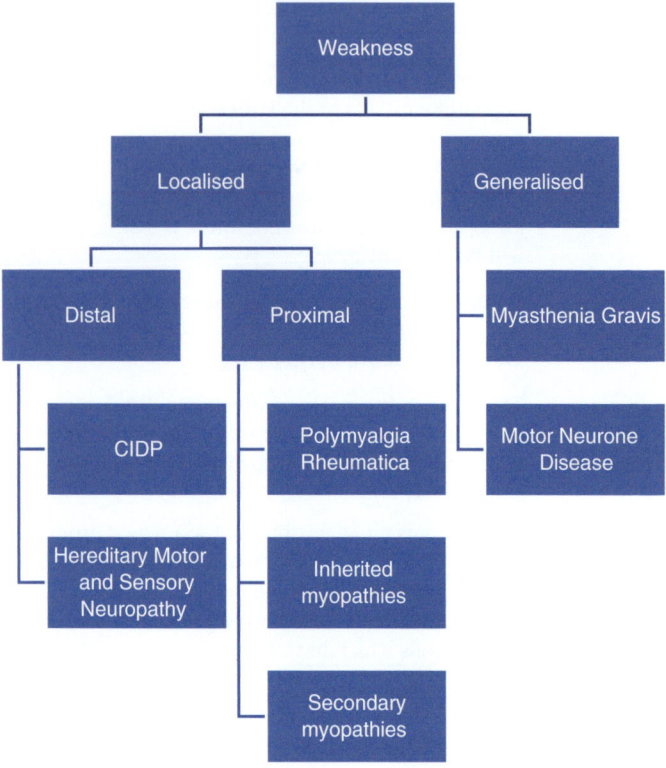

Figure 4.3 This flowchart shows the various causes of muscle weakness

Proximal Weakness

1. Polymyalgia Rheumatica is an autoimmune condition which leads to muscle inflammation. Although it does not cause muscle weakness, the pain and stiffness in the proximal muscles can affect a patient's ability to function. It is diagnosed based on clinical history and raised inflammatory markers on a blood test. There is a close association between polymyalgia rheumatica and temporal arteritis

(mentioned above), therefore it is always important to ask about eye symptoms.
2. Inherited myopathies include Duchenne muscular dystrophy. This leads to progressive weakness and wasting of the muscles. The proximal muscles in the hip tend to be affected earlier on.
3. Secondary myopathies include those which are secondary to endocrinological conditions such as an underactive thyroid or Cushing's disease.

Motor Neurone Disease

Motor neurone disease is a group of diseases which result in destruction to the motor neurons. It can cause both upper and lower motor neuron symptoms. There are no sensory symptoms. There are four main types of motor neurone disease:

(a) Amyotrophic lateral sclerosis—symptoms of this include fasciculations, muscle cramps and weakness. Individuals may trip or fall easily or may be unable to grip anything. It affects both upper and lower motor neurons.
(b) Progressive Bulbar palsy—This presents with difficulty in speaking and swallowing.
(c) Progressive muscular atrophy—This affects the lower motor neurons.
(d) Primary lateral sclerosis—this affects only the upper motor neurons.

Myasthenia Gravis

Myasthenia gravis is a condition which affects the transmission of signals between the nerves and skeletal muscle at the neuromuscular junction (Figure 4.4). A key feature of myasthenia gravis is weakness which is worse after activity and improves after rest. It usually affects the muscles in the face including the muscles around the eye leading to drooping of the eyelid, muscles affecting speech, difficulty swallowing.

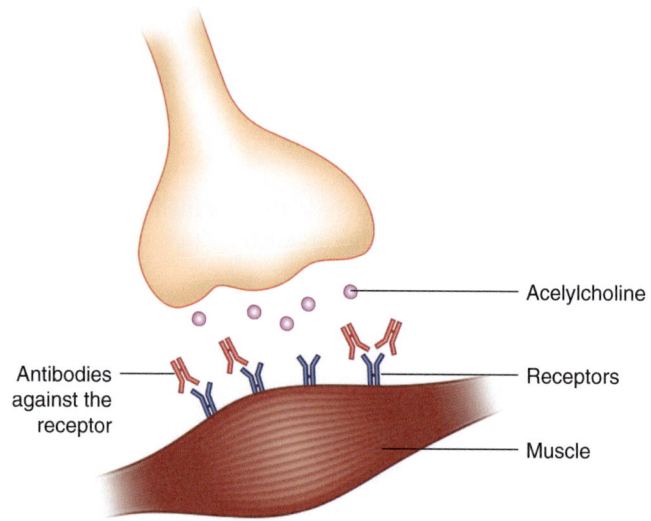

Figure 4.4 This diagram shows the antibodies blocking the acetylcholine receptors in myasthenia gravis. This prevents the neurotransmitter from binding to the receptors

Tremor

A tremor can be a symptom of an underlying condition (Figure 4.5).

Tremors can be divided into resting tremors and action tremors.

- A resting tremor is one which is present when the patient is resting their hands.

    The commonest cause of this is Parkinson's disease. The tremor is said to mimic the action of rolling a pill between your fingers—pill rolling tremor.

    Parkinson's disease presents with

    Bradykinesia
    Rigidity
    And
    Tremor

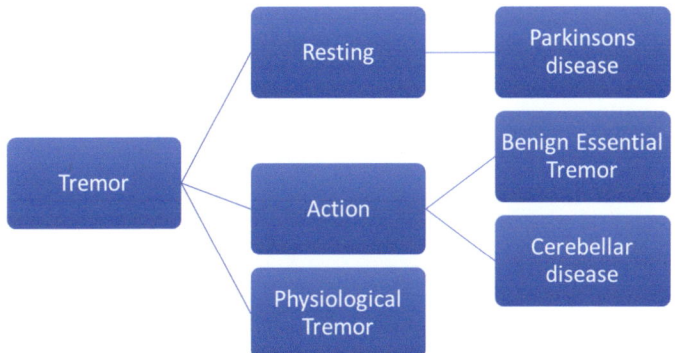

FIGURE 4.5 This flowchart shows the different types of tremor which can develop

(mnemonic: BRAT).

- Intention tremors are a type of action tremor. They are tremors on movement of the arms which exaggerates as the target is approached. The main cause of this includes cerebellar disease. This was discussed in the section on vertigo.
- Benign Essential tremor is a familial condition which causes a tremor usually on movement of the hands. The tremor may begin in one limb and spread to the other limbs over time. Usually patients report that alcohol helps alleviate the tremor. It can be treated with propranolol.
- There are other conditions in which a patient may also have a tremor. These include anxiety and hyperthyroidism. The use of salbutamol can also trigger a fine tremor in a patient. These are sometimes termed exaggerated physiological tremors.

Chapter 5
Musculoskeletal

Joint Pains

Causes of joint pains can be divided up as follows (Table 5.1):

Joint pain is a common presentation. It is important to be able to identify the more serious causes from the less severe.

Patients may present with monoarthritis or polyarthritis. Symptoms can also be acute or chronic.

I will start by discussing the key differences between mechanical and inflammatory arthritis.

I will then discuss key differentials of a single hot swollen joint as this may be an emergency.

Inflammatory Vs Mechanical Joint Pains

Rheumatological Causes

The rheumatological causes of arthritis are due to inflammation of the joint. The patients may have other autoimmune conditions such as type 1 diabetes, thyroid disease or inflammatory bowel disease.

A key symptom in inflammatory arthritis is stiffness. Often the stiffness is worse in the morning and lasts over 30 minutes. The pain tends to be worse after inactivity (in contrast to osteoarthritis).

TABLE 5.1 Table showing common causes of joint pains

Rheumatological causes	Metabolic causes	Orthopaedic causes	Infectious causes
– Rheumatoid arthritis – Sero-negative arthritis (Reactive arthritis, psoriatic arthritis)	– Gout – Pseudogout	– Osteoarthritis – Fractures – Sprains	– Septic arthritis

- Rheumatoid arthritis tends to affect smaller joints (typically the hands). The patient may have positive rheumatoid factor antibodies or anti citrullinated protein antibodies (CCP).
- Seronegative arthritis is arthritis without the positive antibodies which you get with rheumatoid arthritis. It includes:
  - Psoriatic arthritis can occur in patients with a history of psoriasis. Sometimes the arthritis symptoms can precede the development of the skin changes in psoriasis.
  - Enteric arthritis—this is associated with inflammatory bowel disease.
  - Reactive arthritis—this is triggered by an infection (usually STI's or GI infections). It causes joint pains and swelling, and can also cause visual symptoms as well.

Orthopaedic Causes

Osteoarthritis is a very common cause of joint pains. The definition of osteoarthritis is joint pain caused by degeneration of the cartilage. This can occur as we get older and is common in the weight bearing joints such as knees and hips. It can also occur in the small joints of the hand. Other risk factors are increased body mass index and joint injury.

The main symptom of osteoarthritis is pain and stiffness. The stiffness is not as pronounced as that of inflammatory

TABLE 5.2 This table shows the important differential diagnoses in a patient with a single hot swollen joint

Diagnosis	Key features
Gout	Usually affects the large toe. Sudden onset pain and swelling. It occurs due to build-up of uric acid crystals in the joint. It is treated with NSAIDs or colchicine. Excess alcohol intake is a risk factor for gout.
Reactive arthritis	This is arthritis triggered by GI infections or STI's (like chlamydia and gonorrhoea). A common site is inflammation of the knee joint.
Septic arthritis	There may be a history of a wound or skin infection e.g. cellulitis, from where the arthritis originates. Symptoms include a hot red swollen joint, inability to move joint as well as systemic symptoms such as a fever. There will be raised inflammatory markers—WCC and CRP
Fracture	Usually there is a history of injury or an accident. There is sudden onset swelling with difficulty moving or using the joint. It is diagnosed with an X-ray.

arthritis (i.e. it is not there in the morning and lasts less than 30 minutes). The pain is worse when using the joint and improves with rest. This is in contrast to inflammatory arthritis which is worse after rest.

Monoarthritis

It is important to accurately assess the patient with a single hot swollen joint (Table 5.2). The main differential to rule out is a septic joint as this is a surgical emergency.

Back Pain

Back pain is a common presenting complaint you see in general practice and the emergency department.

TABLE 5.3 This table demonstrates the causes of back pain

Mechanical/ orthopaedic	Rheumatological	Infective	Malignant
– Slipped disc – Sciatica – Lumbar canal stenosis	– Ankylosing spondylitis – Psoriatic arthritis	– Discitis – Pott's disease in TB	– Bony metastasis – Myeloma

There are many causes of back pain (Table 5.3). Just like joint pains this can be divided as follows:

Mechanical/Orthopaedic

This is a very common cause of back pain.

- A slipped disc can occur after heavy lifting. The intervertebral disc herniates out and can compress some of the nerves surrounding it.
- Sciatica is a condition in which the sciatic nerve is irritated on its route from the lower back to the legs. It causes shooting pains down the leg.
- Lumbar canal stenosis is narrowing of the spinal canal often secondary to age related degeneration. It presents with bilateral leg pain worse on walking, similar to claudication. Unlike claudication, the pain improves on bending forwards.

> With any back pain, we worry about cauda equina syndrome. The cauda equina is a group of nerves at the end of the spinal cord. It carries the nerves from the spinal cord to the pelvis and lower limbs. If these are compressed it can lead to permanent damage of these nerves. Symptoms of cauda equina include urinary retention, faecal incontinence, perianal numbness and leg weakness. If a patient has any of these symptoms, they need an urgent MRI to rule out cauda equina.

Rheumatological

Ankylosing spondylitis is a condition which causes inflammation of the spine and the sacroiliac joints. Over time, the inflammation can cause fusion of the joints in the spine. Ankylosing spondylitis presents with lower back pain and stiffness that is worse after a period of prolonged rest and improves with movement (like other rheumatological conditions). It tends to affect younger individuals under the age of 45.

Infective

Discitis is a condition caused by infection of the intervertebral disc. It presents with localised back pain associated with other symptoms of infection such as fever and night sweats.

Risk factors for discitis would be any condition that can cause an immunodeficiency. Intravenous drug users are also at higher risk of this.

Pott's disease is a type of discitis caused by tuberculosis.

Malignant

Certain cancers can metastasize to the spine. This causes back pain associated with the other cancer red flags such as weight loss, night sweats and loss of appetite. The patient may also have symptoms of the primary tumour. Cancers that are known to metastasize to the spine include:

- Lung
- Prostate
- Breast

Myeloma is a specific type of haematological cancer which can also present with back pain. It is caused by an increase in the number of plasma cells in the bloodstream. The symptoms are nonspecific and include bony pains, increased bleeding/bruising, lethargy, pathological fractures (fracture with no or minimum trauma). These patients develop kidney disease and high calcium levels.

> **Lina is a 67 year old** lady who presented with thoracic back pain. The pain was did not radiate anywhere else. She had also been to see one of my colleague with right sided leg pain. She was feeling weak and tired, but did not have any obvious weight loss. I decided to arrange some blood tests for her weakness. The results came back fairly unremarkable except for an unexplained normocytic anaemia. She was referred to haematology as I could not find any other explanation for her symptoms. She was eventually diagnosed with multiple myeloma. It is important to think about myeloma as a possible cause of unexplained bony pains. Patients may also have an abnormal renal function and raised calcium on their blood tests. A good mnemonic to remember the symptoms and signs of myeloma is CRAB
>
> hyperCalcaemia
> abnormal Renal function
> Anaemia
> Bony pains

Chapter 6
Other

Leg Swelling

Leg swelling is a fairly common presenting complaint. The causes of leg swelling varies, depending on whether it is bilateral or unilateral.

Bilateral Leg Swelling

1. A common cause of bilateral leg swelling is heart failure, more specifically right heart failure. The heart is unable to pump the blood effectively leading to a backlog of fluid on the right side. The swelling manifests as pitting oedema (pressing a finger on the swollen area leaves an imprint). It improves when the legs are elevated. It would be important to ask about all the other heart failure symptoms we discussed earlier.
2. As well as heart failure, any other organ failure which can lead to fluid overload will also cause leg swelling. This includes liver failure and renal failure.
3. Amlodipine can cause leg swelling as a side effect. It is important to ask about any new drugs initiated recently when taking a history.

4. Varicose veins cause pooling of the blood as the valves in the veins do not function properly. Varicose veins can affect one or both legs.

Unilateral Leg Swelling

1. One of the most important differentials to rule out in a patient with unilateral leg swelling is a deep vein thrombosis. Deep vein thrombosis occurs when there is a clot within the vein. The symptoms include a swollen, red, painful calf. It tends to occur quite suddenly. On examination, the calf is tender and firm to touch. It is important to treat a DVT immediately as there is a risk of the clot breaking off and going into the lung (pulmonary embolism).
2. Another cause of unilateral leg swelling is cellulitis. This is an infection of the skin, and is usually triggered by a cut or bite to the skin. The cardinal symptom is spreading erythema of the skin. In addition, the skin is warm to touch and it may be slightly tender as well. It is treated with a course of antibiotics such as flucloxacillin.
3. Lymphoedema can also cause unilateral swelling of the limbs. Lymphoedema is swelling underneath the skin when there is a disruption to the lymphatic drainage system. This may be congenital or following radiotherapy treatment for cancer which can scar the lymph nodes and block the drainage.
4. Pelvic mass—Pelvic masses can compress the vasculature causing fluid build up in one leg.
5. Varicose veins can sometimes affect only one leg.

Malia

Malia was the last patient on my list on a Friday afternoon. She came is feeling dizzy and complaining of leg swelling. She had been to A + E 2 days ago and was told she had anxiety. She looked quite upset and anxious. Her heart rate was high and she did have new onset oedema. I sent her back to hospital as I wasn't quite sure what her diagnosis was. A few days later, I received a discharge letter which stated that she was diagnosed with nephrotic syndrome. She had protein and blood on her urine dip. This was an important learning point for me: to always do a urine dip in a patient with new onset leg swelling.

Lumps and Bumps

There are many different causes of skin lumps. The commonest ones you will see are:

1. Lymphadenopathy—these are enlarged lymph nodes. We have lymph nodes at various points in our body and they help fight infection. If we have an acute infection, it is not uncommon for the lymph nodes to become enlarged and tender. Common sites of lymphadenopathy are the cervical nodes in the neck which often react to upper respiratory infections. We also have lymph nodes in the groin which can increase in size in response to an abdominal infection.
2. Thyroid nodules/lumps—the thyroid gland is situated at the base of the neck below the cricoid cartilage. An enlarged thyroid is known as a goitre and is often a symptom of a patient with an overactive thyroid gland.
3. Lipoma—there are benign lumps of fat which form under the skin. They are usually mobile and smooth to touch.
4. Sebaceous cysts—these form in hair bearing areas of the body. It occurs due to blocked hair follicles. They are dome shaped and have a punctum in the middle. They can become infected, which results in them becoming red, warm and painful.

A good way to assess your understanding of common presenting complaints is to write down all the possible causes. I have prepared these tables which you can photocopy and use as many times as you want. In the gaps try and think of all the possible diagnoses which could cause the symptoms.

Cardio/Respiratory

Acute chest pain	Chronic chest pain
Acute shortness of breath	Chronic shortness of breath
Cough	Wheeze

Acute chest pain – MI/angina – Arrhythmia – PE – Pneumothorax	Chronic chest pain – Angina – Reflux/heartburn
Acute shortness of breath – PE – Pneumothorax – Acute exacerbation of COPD/asthma – MI – Arrhythmia	Chronic shortness of breath – Heart failure – COPD – Asthma – Interstitial lung disease
Cough – Pneumonia – Heart failure – Reflux – Post nasal drip – Ace inhibitor	Wheeze – Exacerbation of asthma/COPD – Heart failure (cardiac wheeze)

Answer 1

This shows the common cardiorespiratory presenting complaints and possible differentials.

Neurological Histories

Acute headache	Chronic headache
Acute weakness	Chronic weakness
Tremor	Numbness and tingling
Abnormal gait	Visual loss
Seizure	

Acute headache
Meningitis
Subarachnoid haemorrhage
Glaucoma
Temporal arteritis
Malignant hypertension

Chronic headache
Migraine
Cluster headache
Tension headache
Analgesia overuse headache

Acute weakness
Stroke
Flare of multiple sclerosis
Guillain Barre syndrome

Chronic weakness
Muscular dystrophies
Multiple sclerosis
CIDP
Motor/ sensory neuropathies

Tremor
Parkinson's disease
Cerebellar disease
Benign essential tremor
Salbutamol use
Anxiety

Numbness and tingling
Peripheral neuropathy/ mononeuropathy
Anxiety
Multiple sclerosis
Peripheral vascular disease

Seizure	*Visual loss*
Epilepsy	Scleritis/ iritis
Hypoglycaemia	Acute glaucoma
Electrolyte abnormalities	Amaurosis fugax
Encephalitis	

Answer 2

This shows the common neurological presenting complaints and possible differentials.

Abdominal Histories

Acute abdominal pain	Chronic abdominal pain
Diarrhoea	Constipation
Vomiting	PR bleeding
Jaundice	

Acute abdominal pain	*Chronic abdominal pain*
Cholecystitis	Coeliac disease
Pancreatitis	Inflammatory bowel disease
Appendicitis	IBS
Gastroenteritis	Bowel cancer
wwAcute bowel obstruction	Gynaecological pathology
Ovarian cyst accident	

Diarrhoea	*Constipation*
Gastroenteritis	Bowel obstruction
Inflammatory bowel disease	Coeliac disease
Bowel cancer	IBS
	Bowel cancer
	Ovarian pathology

Vomiting	*PR bleeding*
Gastroenteritis	Haemorrhoids/ anal fissure
Pregnancy	Malena (bleeding ulcer)
Pancreatitis	Bowel cancer
Bowel obstruction	Inflammatory bowel disease

Jaundice
Liver disease
Haemolytic anaemia

Answer 3

This shows the common abdominal presenting complaints and possible differentials.

Rheum/Ortho Histories

Acute back pain	Chronic back pain
Acute arthritis	Chronic arthritis

Acute back pain	*Chronic back pain*
Slipped disc	Sciatica
Discitis	Ankylosing spondylitis
Fracture	Bony mets
	Myeloma

Acute arthritis	*Chronic arthritis*
Septic arthritis	Rheumatoid arthritis
Gout	Osteoarthritis
Reactive arthritis	Seronegative arthritis

Answer 4

This shows the common musculoskeletal presenting complaints and possible differentials.

Cases to Practice

Practicing is the most important way to improve your history taking skills.

I have included many different cases for you to practice with your peers. You can use this book to guide you through the questions you need to ask. Feel free to adapt the histories or change some of the facts. These are only there to guide you and inspire you when you practise with your friends.

Case 1

Instructions for the candidate:

> You are an FY1 doctor in accident and emergency. You are about to see Mr. John Dorking, a 55 year old man who has presented with breathlessness.
> Please take a history and discuss your differential diagnoses.

Instructions for the actor:

> HPC: You are Mr. Dorking, a 55 year old man who has suddenly developed pain on the right side of his chest. The pain is sharp and worse on breathing in. You are unable to walk very far—just a few minutes—before you feel breathless. You have no cough and no fever. The pain began this morning and woke you up from sleep. You have never experienced any pain like this

before. You have also been feeling slightly clammy. The pain does not get worse on lying down, it is constant whatever position you are in. You recently travelled to Australia for business and have taken an 18 hour flight. You felt fine initially, but over the last 2 days you have had some pain in your right leg which you thought was due to a muscle pull

PMH: You have recently been told that you have diabetes and started some treatment. You think your cholesterol may be high.

Drugs: You have no allergies. You take metformin.

Fhx: your father had angina when he was older. Your mother suffered from a DVT when she was young. She thought this was due to a medication she was taking.

Shx: You have never had any problems with breathing despite being a smoker for 20 years. You smoke 20 cigarettes a day. You drink 8 pints on the weekend when you go to the pub. You live on your own in a flat and work as a businessman.

ICE: You are worried about the pain as you have never experienced anything like this. You are frightened and would like to have a chest X-ray. You are also stressed as you have an important meeting tomorrow and would like to get this sorted so you can go back to work.

Instructions for the examiner:

Criteria	Marks awarded
Elicits the presenting complaint (1)	
Asks the following—pleuritic pain, shortness of breath, leg swelling, recent travel (1 mark each – max 4)	
Asks about past medical history (1)	
Asks about drug history (1)	
Asks about family history (1)	
Asks about social history -MUST ask about smoking to get this point (1)	

Elicits ICE (1 mark)

Total (max 10)

Discussion

Top of the list of differential diagnoses would be a pulmonary embolism given the presentation (pleuritic chest pain, leg pain? DVT, shortness of breath, long haul flight).

Case 2

Instructions for the candidate:

> You are a junior doctor working in GP. Please take history from Sarah, a 20 year old female. Following the history, please present your findings and discuss your differential diagnoses.

Instructions for the actor:

> HPC: You are Sarah, a 20 year old female, who has been suffering with constipation and diarrhoea for the last year on and off. You occasionally get some cramps in your stomach. You haven't changed your diet in the last year, however you do feel worse after eating carbohydrate based foods.
>
> Your main symptoms are diarrhoea and constipation. It seems to fluctuate. You have never noticed any blood in your stool. You have had a small amount of weight loss, but your appetite is the same. You used to enjoy pizza, but now can't seem to have any which upsets you.
>
> PMH: You do not have any other medical problems. You have been taking the COCP for 2 years without any problems. You are in a stable relationship and are not stressed.
>
> FHX: You have a family history of grave's disease. Your mum was diagnosed with this 10 years ago. She presented with diarrhoea which is why you would like a blood test to check your thyroid function.
>
> SHX: You are studying in university and live with your boyfriend. You do not smoke but you drink 2–3 cocktails on the weekend.

You are concerned that you might have an overactive thyroid. You would like some blood tests.

ICE: You are getting embarrassed with your symptoms as you have had to rush to the toilet a few times when out with friends.

Instructions for the examiner:

Criteria	Marks awarded
Elicits the presenting complaint (1)	
Asks the following—constipation and diarrhoea, link to gluten containing foods (1 mark each – max 3)	
Asks about red flags: Blood in the stool, weight loss, loss of appetite (3)	
Asks about past medical history & drug history (1)	
Asks about family history (1)	
Asks about social history (1)	
Elicits ICE (1 mark)	
Total (max 10)	

The main differential diagnosis here would be coeliac disease due to the link to gluten containing foods. It would also be worth checking for an overactive thyroid as well as a inflammatory bowel disease, as there is a family history of autoimmune disease. Although IBS is a possibility, it is a diagnosis of exclusion.

Case 3

Instructions for the candidate:

You are an FY1 working in the accident and emergency department. Please take a history from Mr. O'Brien, a 65 year old gentleman, who has been brought in by his wife.

80 Chapter 6. Other

Instructions for the actor:

HPC: Your name is John O'brien and you are a 65 year old retired banker.

For the last 2 days you have been feeling bloated and constipated. This morning you woke up feeling sick and have been vomiting up large amounts. You cannot keep anything down. You look as though you are pregnant. If asked you would describe the vomit as greenish in colour. There is no blood. Only if asked, let the doctor know that you have not passed wind since yesterday.

You have some generalised pain and overall are feeling quite weak. You do not have a fever.

PMH: You are otherwise quite well.

Dhx: You take a statin for cholesterol and some blood pressure tablets. You do not have any allergies.

Fhx: you cannot recall anything of note

Shx: You live with your wife who has been very concerned. You used to work for a bank and recently retired. You are looking forward to going travelling in a few months to visit your children. You drink socially but you don't smoke.

ICE: You think you are just constipated and would like some laxatives to open your bowels

Instructions for the examiner:

Criteria	Marks awarded
Elicits the presenting complaint (1)	
Asks the following—constipation, vomiting, bloating (1 mark each – max 3)	
Asks about red flags: Haematemesis, not passing wind (2)	
Asks about past medical history & drug history (1)	
Asks about family history (1)	
Asks about social history (1)	

Elicits ICE (1 mark)
Total (max 10)

The main differential diagnosis here would be bowel obstruction. The commonest causes of bowel obstruction include the following

- small bowel obstruction: adhesions and hernias
- large bowel obstruction: malignancy

Case 4

Instructions for candidate:

> You are a GP trainee doing a routine clinic. Your next patient is Mr. Marcus Webster, a 55 year old man. Please take a history and present your findings.

Instructions for the actor:

> HPC: You are Marcus Webster, a 55 year old man who has developed worsening back pain over the last week. You have suffered from back pain on and off before this, but over the last week your symptoms have worsened. The pain is in the lower back and there is some shooting pain down your right leg. There is no numbness or tingling. If asked, mention that the pain was triggered by some heavy lifting of furniture you did last week.

> The pain is not improving with ibuprofen and a hot water bottle. Only if asked, inform the doctor that you have some problems passing urine—you are finding it more difficult to pass urine since yesterday. Your bowels are ok.

> PMH: You are otherwise well. You take metformin for diabetes and a statin for your cholesterol. You do not have any drug allergies.

> FHx: There is no family history of note.

> Shx: You work as a builder and recently had to do a lot of heavy lifting at work which triggered the pain. You have

been unable to work for the last week which has reduced your income as you are self employed. You are keen to get this fixed fast so that you can get back to work.

You live with your wife and your teenage son. They are very supportive.

ICE: You think you may have a slipped disc and would like to be referred to physiotherapy. You would also like some stronger painkillers. You are shocked when the doctor tells you that you need to go to hospital but agree to do so as you understand the urgency of the situation.

Instructions for examiner:

Criteria	Marks awarded
Elicits the presenting complaint (1)	
Asks the following—shooting pain down the leg, no numbness and tingling, triggered by heavy lifting (1 mark each – max 3)	
Asks about red flags: Problems with bladder and bowels (2)	
Asks about past medical history & drug history (1)	
Asks about family history (1)	
Asks about social history (1)	
Elicits ICE (1 mark)	
Total (max 10)	

The main differential diagnosis here is cauda equina syndrome due to the new onset urinary symptoms. This patient will need to be referred to accident and emergency for an urgent MRI lumbar spine. This is an emergency and therefore the candidate would not be able to pass the station unless they mention this.

Case 5

Instructions for the candidate:

You are a core medical trainee in accident and emergency. Your next patient is Felicity, a 23 year old female who has come in with palpitations. Please take a history and discuss your differential diagnoses.

Instructions for the actor:

HPC: You are Felicity Smith, a 23 year old student who has had a sensation of her heart pounding in her chest for the last 20 mins. You have had this occur a few times before, but it normally lasts 30 seconds. This time it is much longer. You have a slight tightness in your chest and are feeling dizzy. You feel that your heart rate is irregular.

These episodes have been happening sporadically for the last few months. You have not noticed anything in particular. You have never collapsed If asked, mention that you have also noticed weight loss and you have been feeling more anxious than usual. Your friends also commented that your neck looks fatter than usual.

PMH: You are normally fit and well. You do not take any medications.

Fhx: With regards to your family history, your mother was diagnosed with Grave's disease 15 years ago.

Shx: You are studying to be a dentist and are renting a flat with your friends. You do not smoke and drink socially.

ICE: you are very concerned about your heart and are worried that it will stop working properly. You had a friend who had a cardiac arrest playing sports and this is really worrying you.

Chapter 6. Other

Instructions for the examiner:

Criteria	Marks awarded
Elicits the presenting complaint (1)	
Asks the following – duration of palpitations, chest pain, dizziness, irregular heart beat, weight loss (1 mark each – max 5)	
Asks about past medical history & drug history (1)	
Asks about family history (1)	
Asks about social history (1)	
Elicits ICE (1 mark)	
Total (max 10)	

This patient is suffering from an arrhythmia. As she mentioned that her heart beat is irregular this is likely atrial fibrillation. Given her symptoms of weight loss, anxiety and the family history of Grave's it is likely that the atrial fibrillation is secondary to thyrotoxicosis.

Case 6

Instructions for the candidate:

> You are a GP working in a remote practice. Your next patient is a 65 year old female. Please take a history and discuss your differential diagnosis.

Instructions for the actor:

> HPC: You are Mrs. Theresa O'conner, a 70 year old female who has been experiencing some abdominal discomfort and bloating for the last few months. You have also had some days where you are very constipated and some days when you have loose stool.
>
> The bloating is worse after eating, but you haven't noticed any specific foods which trigger this. The pain is in the lower abdomen. It is like a dull ache.

You haven't lost any weight, if anything you think you are looking fuller around the belly. You are surprised by this as you have been eating much less recently. This is because the bloating makes you feel nauseous. You have not noticed any blood in your stool.

PMH: You have a background of diverticular disease which was diagnosed 10 years ago. The main symptom of this is the occasional pain on your left side associated with diarrhoea, but it normally clears up with antibiotics quite quickly. This feels different.

Medication: You take a statin for your cholesterol and some vitamin D tablets.

Fhx: Your mother and aunt had breast cancer. If you are asked if they were tested for the BRCA gene, mention that you do not know.

Shx: You are a retired school teacher. You retired last year. You live with your husband and dog.

ICE: You aren't sure what this is. You wanted to discuss if this could be related to your diverticular disease.

Instructions for the examiner:

Criteria	Marks awarded
Elicits the presenting complaint (1)	
Asks the following—bloating, change in bowel habits (1 mark each – max 2)	
Asks about red flags—weight loss, loss of appetite, PR bleeding (3)	
Asks about past medical history & drug history (1)	
Asks about family history (1)	
Asks about social history (1)	
Elicits ICE (1 mark)	
Total (max 10)	

This is a vague history. The differentials would include both bowel cancer and ovarian cancer. The patient has a change in bowel habit. In an older person this should prompt you to think about bowel cancer. In women, this can also be a symptom of ovarian cancer and a CA-125 should be included in the investigations. The family history of breast cancer and the bloating/ weight gain around the abdomen would be more suggestive of an ovarian malignancy.

Case 7

Instructions for the candidate:

> You are a GP who is visiting Mr. Daniels, a 75 year old man who has suddenly become breathless in the last 2 days.

Instructions for the actor:

> HPC: You are coughing a lot of green mucus and have noticed a funny noise in your chest when you breathe in. You can't check your temperature, however you think you may have a fever as you have been feeling hot and cold.

> If asked, you have some tightness across your chest and it hurts when you start to cough. You are feeling very breathless and can only walk a few minutes before having to stop. Normally you can walk on the flat for up to 20 min before you feel out of breath.

> You have not coughed up any blood.

> PMH: You have a diagnosis of COPD for which you take some inhalers. They usually help, but at the moment, they don't seem to making much difference to how you are feeling. You also have some high blood pressure and take ramipril for this.

> You have no known drug allergies.

> Shx: You live by yourself in a ground floor flat. You are normally very independent although it takes you much longer to walk around and do your errands. YOu do not have any carers and you have no family nearby.

You think you may have a chest infection and would like antibiotics.

Instructions for examiner:

Criteria	Marks awarded
Elicits the presenting complaint (1)	
Asks the following -fever, mucous, wheeze (1 mark each – max 3)	
Asks about red flags: Shortness of breath, chest pain, haemoptysis (1 mark each – max 3)	
Asks about past medical history (1)	
Asks about social history -MUST ask about smoking to get this point (1)	
Elicits ICE (1 mark)	
Total (max 10)	

This patient has an infective exacerbation of his COPD. He will need to be assessed to check his oxygen levels and is likely to need both antibiotics and steroids to treat his exacerbation.

Case 8

Instructions for the candidate:

You are an FY1 in A + E. Your next patient is Mr. Lucas, a 35 year old man who has come in with abdominal pain.

Instructions for the actor:

HPC: You are Marc Lucas, a 35 year old investment banker who has intense epigastric pain. This is the worst pain you have ever experienced in your life. The pain is a sharp pain and goes all the way from the front to the back. You have also been vomiting since early morning. Your vomit is a green colour. There is no blood in your vomit. You do not have any diarrhoea. You do not have a fever, although you are feeling quite hot and sweaty. You have never experienced anything like this before.

You have not been able to keep any fluids down. You last passed urine a few hours ago.

PMH: you are fit and well. You do not take any medications

Penicillin allergy

SHX: You live by yourself. You work as an investment banker in the city. Your job is high pressured and you have to entertain clients a lot. You probably drink about 30 units a week. You know this is a lot, but you get carried away. You don't smoke.

ICE: You initially thought this was reflux and tried to take gaviscon. You are in a lot of pain and would like some strong painkillers.

Instructions for examiner:

Criteria	Marks awarded
Elicits the presenting complaint (1)	
Asks the following -radiation of pain, vomiting, fever, diarrhoea (1 mark each – max 4)	
Asks about red flags: Haematemesis, urine output (2 marks)	
Asks about past medical history (1)	
Asks about social history -MUST ask about alcohol to get this point (1)	
Elicits ICE (1 mark)	
Total (max 10)	

This patient likely has acute pancreatitis secondary to high alcohol consumption. Investigations should include a serum amylase level which is raised in pancreatitis.

Case 9

Instructions for the candidate:

> You are a GP. Your next patient is Robert, a 39 year old man who has presented with some back pain. Please take a history and discuss your differential diagnosis.

Instructions for the actor:

> HPC: You are Robert Grove, a 39 year old accountant who has been noticing some lower back pain for a few months. It is usually worse first thing in the morning and you also find it really hard to get out of bed. Once you are out of bed, you usually start to feel a little better and the pain improves during the day. However you do feel stiff when you need to get up out of your chair at work. You do not have any shooting pain down the back of your leg. You do not have any problems passing urine and have no numbness in your perineal region.
>
> There was no history of trauma at the time you started having the back pain. You also do not have pain in any of your other joints.
>
> PMH: You have psoriasis which is currently well controlled. You occasionally need to use steroid creams in the winter when it flares up slightly.
>
> No known drug allergies
>
> Fhx: psoriasis and diabetes.
>
> Shx: You work as an accountant and live in a house with your wife and two kids. You are managing okay but occasionally need to take painkillers for the pain.
>
> ICE: You are cornered that you may have a slipped disc. You think you might need some physiotherapy.

Chapter 6. Other

Instructions for the examiner:

Criteria	Marks awarded
Elicits the presenting complaint (1)	
Asks the following—when the pain is worse, stiffness, shooting pain down the leg (3 marks)	
Asks about red flags: Difficulty passing urine/bowel, perineal numbness(2 marks)	
Asks about past medical history and family history (2)	
Asks about social history (1)	
Elicits ICE (1 mark)	
Total (max 10)	

The symptoms of early morning stiffness and improved symptoms following movement are suggestive of inflammatory arthritis. The differentials would be ankylosing spondylitis or psoriatic arthritis.

Case 10

Instructions for the candidate:

You are a GP trainee working in an urgent care centre. Your next patient is Angela, a 25 year old female who has come in with some tingling in her legs. Please take a history and discuss your differential diagnoses.

Instructions for the actor:

HPC: Your name is Angela Smith and you are an actress. Over the last few weeks, you have had some tingling in your right leg. It feels a little weaker to move as well, but you are still able to walk with difficulty. You do not have any back pain. You had something similar in your left arm a few months ago, which settled in a few days. You have not injured yourself. You do not have a headache. If asked, mention that you had some problems with your vision last year. It was painful for 2–3 days. You thought you may have conjunctivitis. This has not happened again since last year.

PMH: You have some eczema. You are otherwise fit and well.

You do not take any regular medication and have an allergy to ibuprofen.

Fhx: Your aunty has recently been diagnosed with a brain tumour. She had some tingling in her arms as well.

Shx: You live on your own in an apartment. There is no lift which makes it harder to go out of your flat when you have the symptoms.

You smoke 5 cigarettes a day and drink very rarely.

ICE: You are worried that you may also have a brain tumour and would like to be referred for a brain scan.

Instructions for the examiner:

Criteria	Marks awarded
Elicits the presenting complaint (1)	
Asks the following—any other epidodes, asks about back pain, asks about trauma, asks about headaches (5 marks)	
Asks about past medical history and family history (2)	
Asks about social history (1)	
Elicits ICE (1 mark)	
Total (max 10)	

The episodic history is suggestive of multiple sclerosis. The visual symptoms are likely to have been due to optic neuritis.

Chapter 7
Gynaecology

Abnormalities of the Menstrual Cycle

Menorrhagia

Menorrhagia is the term used for 'heavy menstrual bleeding'.

When taking a Menorrhagia history try and quantify how much blood loss there is. An easy way to do this is to ask how often a woman needs to change her pad or tampon and if it is soaking through. You can also ask them to compare it to what their normal level of bleeding is. If a woman has always had heavy bleeding since they were a teenager, the cause of this is likely to be different then if the woman developed menorrhagia later in life.

If a woman has Menorrhagia, it is important to consider the following causes:

Gynaecological Causes

1. Dysfunctional uterine bleeding—this is the term used to describe heavy bleeding of an unknown cause. It tends to be common in the first few years post menarche and the last few years prior to menopause.
2. Endometriosis—this describes a condition in which the endometrial lining extends beyond the uterus. The symp-

toms include painful, heavy periods as well as deep pain during intercourse and chronic pelvic pain. Patients may also complain of abnormal bowel symptoms during their periods. It is diagnosed with a laparoscopy.
3. Adenomyosis—this is when the endometrial lining embeds deeper into the myometrium of the womb. It can also present with heavy, painful periods.
4. Fibroids—these are benign growths in the womb. They can cause both intermenstrual bleeding and heavy/ painful bleeding. If they are large enough they can even cause endometrial distortion as well as bloating, back pain and urinary symptoms.
5. Polyps—these are benign tumours in the uterus. Like fibroids, they can also cause intermenstrual bleeding.
6. IUD—The copper coil (intrauterine device) is a non-hormonal contraceptive. It can cause the period to become much more heavy and painful. This is in contrast to the IUS (mirena coil) which is a hormonal coil. This results in lighter/ absent periods.

Systemic Causes

1. Clotting dysfunction—any abnormalities in clotting factors or platelet levels may cause heavy periods. An example of this would be a woman with Von Wilibrands disease (a haematological condition that affects blood clotting).
2. Thyroid abnormalities—underactive or overactive thyroid function can affect the amount of menstrual bleeding.

Dysmenorrhea

This goes hand in hand with Menorrhagia and often the two symptoms coincide.

Often pain which starts at the onset of a period is normal and is not usually associated with any underlying pathology (primary dysmenorrhea). This is especially true if the woman has experienced this type of pain from menarche (the onset of her periods).

However if the pain precedes the onset of the period (secondary dysmenorrhea), this is indicative of underlying pathology. Conditions which can cause secondary dysmenorrhea include the following. You will notice a lot of overlap between the causes of dysmenorrhea and menorrhagia.

Gynaecological Causes

1. Endometriosis/ adenomyosis—see above
2. Fibroids/polyps—see above
3. pelvic inflammatory disease—This is due to infection in the cervix and uterus. It is often due to upward extension of the same organisms which cause sexually transmitted infections (STI's). Symptoms include pelvic pain, foul smelling discharge and deep dyspareunia (pain with intercourse).

Amenorrhea

This is the term given to the absence of periods. There are two main categories of amenorrhea (Table 7.1).

Primary Amenorrhea

This describes the situation when a female (of age 15 years and over) never gets her periods in the first place (failure to reach menarche). This could be due to many reasons.

- Genetic abnormalities—genetic conditions which affect the development of the female reproductive tract will lead to amenorrhea. Examples of this would be Turner's syndrome and Fragile X syndrome. It would be important to ask about any learning or developmental difficulties growing up. It would also be important to take a detailed history about sexual development and puberty. For example

Table 7.1 This table shows the secondary sexual characteristics that develop during puberty

Secondary sexual characteristic to enquire about in a history
Breast development
Widening of hips
Pubic hair growth
Axillary hair growth

there may be a lack of breast development or pubic hair growth.

- Structural abnormalities—If the woman has normal secondary sexual characteristics, structural abnormalities in the uterus may be the cause of the amenorrhea. These would include an imperforate hymen or transverse vaginal septum (Figure 7.1).
- Hormonal abnormalities

  1. Androgen insensitivity syndrome—This is a condition in which a person who is genetically male (XY) is insensitive to androgen and therefore will have female characteristics. However as they have no womb, they will not develop periods.

  2. high prolactin levels—High prolactin levels suppress LH and FSH via the pathway shown below. Therefore anything which causes a raised prolactin will cause amenorrhea. Causes of a raised prolactin include:
     - prolactinoma
     - certain medications such as antipsychotics.

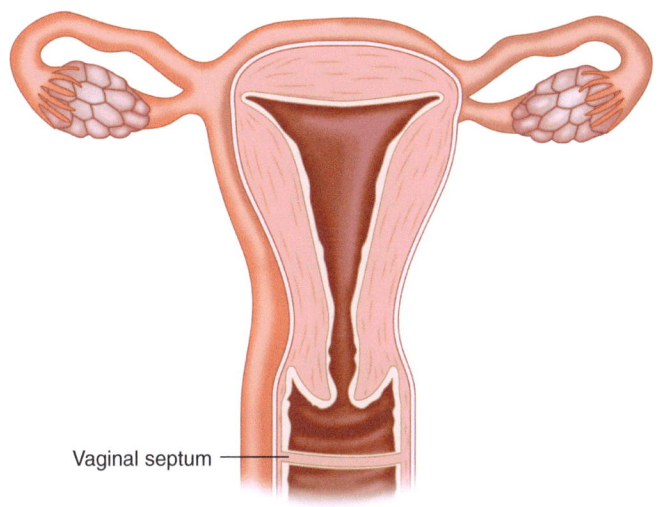

Figure 7.1 This diagram shows a transverse vaginal septum

Secondary Amenorrhea

This is the cessation of periods in a woman who has previously reached menarche. The precise definition is cessation of periods for 3–6 months in a woman with regular periods or 6–12 months in someone with irregular periods.

It's causes include:

- Hormonal abnormalities/ sheehan's syndrome — Ovulation and menstruation are controlled by a hormonal pathway regulated by the hypothalamus. Anything which disrupts this cycle can cause amenorrhea.
- One fairly common cause of hormonal dysregulation is anorexia/weight loss which can disrupt this hormone feedback cycle.
- Another cause is Sheehan's syndrome. This is damage to the pituitary gland from excess blood loss during delivery.

- Other conditions which affect the hypothalamus or pituitary can cause amenorrhea. For example a prolactinoma can disrupt the pathway. The following diagram highlights the hormonal pathway which controls menstruation (Figure 7.2). As you can see, raised prolactin negatively influences the pathway resulting in a reduced production of Leutinizing Hormone (LH) and Follicular Stimulating Hormone (FSH):
- Medications—certain medications cause amenorrhea. For example the contraceptive injection may cause a woman to remain amenorrheic for a while once stopped. Antipsychotics can also cause raised prolactin levels and therefore amenorrhea.
- Polycystic ovarian syndrome—This is a very common cause of amenorrhea in women. It is usually caused by hormonal imbalances in the body which affect FSH and LH.
- There are three main aspects to a diagnosis of polycystic ovaries:

  1. polycystic ovaries on an ultrasound scan
  2. irregular periods or absent periods

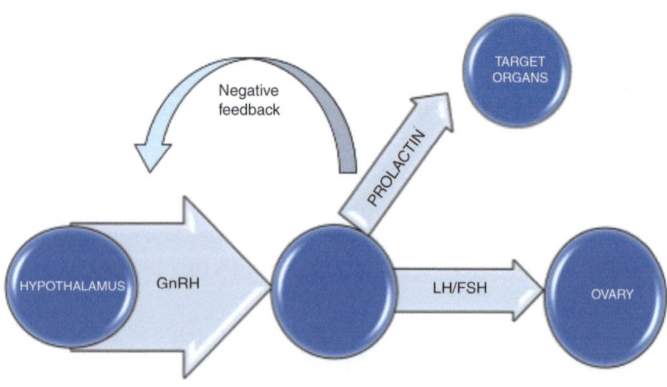

FIGURE 7.2 This diagram demonstrates the negative feedback cycle which controls LH and FSH production

3. hyperandrogenism on blood tests and symptoms of raised androgen levels including abnormal hair growth and acne.

   To be diagnosed with the syndrome, you only need 2 out of 3 of these. Often being overweight can make the symptoms worse and weight loss is always advised.

- Ashermans syndrome — This is the formation of scar tissue in the uterus following instrumentation such as after a surgical termination. This can sometimes impede the flow of blood causing amenorrhea.
- Premature ovarian failure/ menopause — The menopause occurs around the age of 51. It is a natural process in which the ovary stops producing oestrogen and progesterone. In some women, this process occurs earlier than expected, a condition called premature ovarian failure. It is unclear what exactly causes this. It can be genetic or autoimmune.

Abnormal Bleeding Patterns

Intermenstrual Bleeding

This is any bleeding between periods. Sometimes this can be normal and some women spot during ovulation. However other causes include:

- Fibroids/polyps
- Infection — STI's or pelvic inflammatory disease can lead to abnormal bleeding. It is important to take a detailed sexual history, enquire about any new partners as well as any abnormal discharge.
- Pregnancy — some women may bleed during implantation of the embryo — implantation spotting.
- Malignancy — cervical or endometrial malignancies can cause bleeding between periods.

Post-Coital Bleeding

Post-coital bleeding is usually due to cervical pathology. Irritation of the cervix during intercourse triggers the bleeding. Causes of post coital bleeding include.

1. cervical cancer
2. polyps
3. cervicitis (Pelvic Inflammatory Disease)
4. ectropion—this is when the glandular cells in the internal part of the cervix extend outwards, replacing the squamous epithelium. These cells are more fragile and therefore bleed easily. This is caused by hormone changes such as during pregnancy or if a woman is on the Combined contraceptive Pill.

Post-Menopausal Bleeding

Post menopausal bleeding is always assumed to be endometrial cancer until proven otherwise. Therefore this should always be your top differential diagnosis and a woman should always be investigated for this. Other causes include:

1. Polyps
2. Fibroids
3. HRT—hormone replacement therapy can sometimes cause bleeding when a woman first starts using it.
4. Infections—STI's can cause abnormal vaginal bleeding. Always take a sexual history and ask about any new partners.
5. Atrophy of the vagina—this is when the vaginal wall becomes thin and dry following the reduction in oestrogen production with menopause. As a result it can bleed and cause some spotting.

Abnormal Pain

Dyspareunia

This is pain during intercourse. The pain can either be superficial or deep and the causes will vary depending on where the pain is.

Superficial Dyspareunia

This is pain at the entrance of the vagina and is caused by problems at the vulva or lower part of the vagina. These include:

- Skin conditions such as lichen sclerosis can make intercourse much more painful.
- Vaginismus—this is increased muscle contraction around the vulva and vagina during intercourse. This makes penetration much more difficult and is also painful.
- Infections such as thrush
- Atrophic vaginitis secondary to menopause

Deep Dyspareunia

This is pain in the pelvis during intercourse. It usually indicates either

- Endometriosis/ adenomyosis
- Pelvic inflammatory disease—This is infection of the pelvic organs as a result of an STI.

Pelvic Pain

If a patient presents with pelvic pain, this can be due to gynaecological, abdominal or urinary tract pathology. Have a look back at the table in the abdominal chapter to remind yourself of the various causes. I will now discuss the gynaecological causes in more detail. Pelvic pain can be acute or chronic.

Acute Pelvic Pain (Table 7.2)

TABLE 7.2 This table highlights common causes of acute pelvic pain

Suprapubic pain	Right/left iliac fossa
– Pregnancy – pregnancy may cause abnormal cramps in the suprapubic region. – Fibroids – Pelvic inflammatory disease	– Pregnancy – need to consider ectopic pregnancy if there is unilateral pain. – Ovarian cyst accident – ovarian cysts can rupture, bleed and twist which causes pain. – Ovulation pain – this is called Mirtelchmirtz disease and is pain during ovulation.

Chronic Pelvic Pain (Table 7.3)

TABLE 7.3 This table highlights common causes of chronic pelvic pain

Suprapubic pain	right/left iliac fossa pain
Endometriosis Adenomyosis	Ovarian cysts – Large cysts such as dermoid cysts can cause unilateral pain. Ovarian cancers – These present insidiously and can often mimic irritable bowel syndrome. Always consider a diagnosis of ovarian cancer in an older women presenting with bloating and indigestion, especially if she has never experienced this before.

> **Sofia**
>
> Sofia is a 60 year old lady who came to see me with bloating and flatulence after eating. Her symptoms has started a few months ago. She felt that her tummy was looking bigger, and she wasn't able to eat as much as she previously did because of her bloating. She thought there was something wrong with her gut as her friend had recently been diagnosed with irritable bowel syndrome. I performed a series of tests, including blood tests and a stool test. Her Ca-125 ovarian cancer marker was raised and she was referred to gynaecology. She was eventually diagnosed with ovarian cancer. This case was a useful reminder that ovarian cancer can present with gut symptoms, and should always be considered in the differential diagnosis of someone with bloating.

As you can see there is a lot of overlap between the causes of these presenting complaints. To make sure you have understood how common gynaecological conditions present, fill in the table with the symptoms caused by these conditions:

Condition	Symptoms
Endometriosis	
Pelvic inflammatory disease	
Adenomyosis	
Fibroids	

Condition	Symptoms
Endometrial polyps	
Endometrial cancer	
Cervical cancer	
Ovarian cancer	

Example Answers

Condition	Symptoms
Endometriosis	Pelvic pain Severe period pain Menorrhagia Pain during sex
Pelvic inflammatory disease	Pelvic pain Discharge Fever
Adenomyosis	Similar to endometriosis
Fibroids	Pain — may also cause back pain as well Abnormal bleeding Heavy periods

Condition	Symptoms
Endometrial polyps	Intermenstrual bleeding or heavy periods
Endometrial cancer	Intermenstrual or post menopausal bleeding
Cervical cancer	Intermenstrual bleeding or post-coital bleeding
Ovarian cancer	Left or right iliac fossa pain or mass Bloating Indigestion

Answer 5

This shows common gynaecological presenting diagnosis and how they present.

Obstetrics and Gynaecology

When taking an obstetric and gynaecological history it may be important to ask some extra questions in addition to your standard history questions. These questions are about sexual and reproductive health and include:

Gynaecological History

1. How are your periods? Are they regular or irregular? Any pain or heavy bleeding?
2. Do you take contraception or have you taken contraception previously?

3. Are you sexually active? Do you have a regular partner?
4. Any vaginal discharge?
5. Any abnormal bleeding e.g. bleeding between your periods? bleeding after sex?
6. Are you up to date with your smears?

Obstetric History

1. How many times have you been pregnant before?
2. Have you had any miscarriages or terminations?
3. How have your previous deliveries been- c-section/ forceps/ ventousse/ tears?
4. Any complications during your previous pregnancies e.g. pre-eclampsia, obstetric cholestasis?

Obstetric Nomenclature

When describing how many pregnancies a woman has had, you can use the following nomenclature -

- Gravity—this is the total number of pregnancies the woman has had (including terminations and miscarriages).
- Parity—this is the total number of viable pregnancies a woman has had (above 24 weeks gestation)

For example a woman who has had two pregnancies and two children would be G2P2.

If a women had two pregnancies including one miscarriage she would be G2P1 + 1 (the +1 refers to the miscarriage before 24 weeks).

It may not be necessary to ask all of the questions mentioned above, and you can choose which ones to ask depending on the presenting complaint.

Chapter 8
Obstetrics

Abnormal Bleeding during Pregnancy (Table 8.1)

TABLE 8.1 This table shows the possible causes of bleeding during each semester of pregnancy

Early pregnancy	**Second trimester**	**Third trimester**
Miscarriage (within the first 3 months)	Late miscarriage (after 3 months)	Placental abruption—this is when the placenta separates from the uterus wall prior to delivery
Ectopic pregnancy—this is when the embryo implants in the fallopian tube. As it enlarges, it can cause pain, and eventually can cause rupture of the tube.	Placenta praevia—this is a low lying placenta which covers the opening of the cervix. It can lead to painless bleeding after 20 weeks of pregnancy. It is usually diagnosed on an ultrasound scan.	Placenta praevia—this is a low lying placenta which covers the opening of the cervix. It can lead to painless bleeding after 20 weeks of pregnancy. It is usually diagnosed on an ultrasound scan.

© The Author(s), under exclusive license to Springer Nature Switzerland AG 2023
K. Mahbubani, *History Taking in Clinical Practice*, In Clinical Practice, https://doi.org/10.1007/978-3-031-29897-4_8

Abnormal Pain during Pregnancy

Common causes of abdominal pain during pregnancy:

Pain in the first trimester

- Miscarriage—a miscarriage usually presents in the first 12 weeks. It can present with cramps which resemble period pains. Women will also have vaginal bleeding as the uterine contents are removed from the body.
- Ectopic pregnancy—This may present in different ways. Symptoms usually present after 4 weeks when the embryo starts to get bigger. It can present with left or right iliac fossa pain (depending on which side it is). Some women may also have bleeding.
- UTI—pregnant women are more prone to UTIs. They present in a similar way with dysuria and suprapubic pain. It is very important to treat all UTIs in pregnancy as it increases the risk of preterm labour.

Pain in the second/third trimester

- Heartburn—the pressure of the foetus on the stomach can trigger some heartburn.
- Constipation—similar pressure effects secondary to the pregnant uterus can cause women to become constipated and also develop haemorrhoids.
- UTI—UTI's can happen at any stage in pregnancy.
- HELLP syndrome/ preeclampsia—preeclampsia is a condition which occurs in pregnancy resulting in high blood pressure and protein in the urine. It is important to identify this as it can cause complications such as clotting abnormalities and increased risk of stroke and seizures in the mother. It can also affect the growth and development of the baby as it is often associated with reduced blood flow through the placenta.

Symptoms of pre eclampsia include:
 *headache
 *swelling of hands, feet and face

*pain below the ribcage (RUQ pain)
*vomiting

Sometimes pre-eclampsia can develop into HELLP syndrome. This stands for Haemolysis, Elevate Liver Enzymes and Low Platelets. It presents in a similar way to pre-eclampsia and therefore women need close monitoring of their blood tests to ensure they are not anaemic and their liver function tests are normal. HELLP syndrome can be life threatening and often a woman who has developed the condition will be induced early.

– Placental abruption—This describes a process in which the placenta separates from the uterus prior to delivery. It presents with bleeding and pain in the third trimester. Depending on the degree of blood loss, women may need an emergency c-section to treat abruption.
– Labour—most women will go into labour between 37–40 weeks of pregnancy. Labour starts with Braxton Hicks contractions before it becomes much more frequent in active labour.

Itching in Pregnancy

Dermatological Causes

There are a few causes of itchy rashes in pregnancy. These include:

– PUPPS or pruritic urticarial papules and plaques of pregnancy is a condition which causes a red itchy allergic type rash to appear around the belly during the last trimester of pregnancy. It can also spread to other parts of the body. It is a harmless condition.
– Pemphigoid gestationis—This is an autoimmune condition which affects women in mid to late pregnancy. It causes an urticarial rash which eventually can lead to blisters. Unlike PUPPS this can affect the pregnancy and can lead to premature delivery. In a small percentage of pregnancies, the baby may also have skin blisters.

Systemic Causes

The main systemic cause of itching in pregnancy is intrahepatic cholestasis. There is no rash. In this condition, the bile salts leak out into the blood-stream resulting in itching particularly in the palms and soles of the feet. It usually occurs after 24 weeks of gestation. Other symptoms include nausea and tiredness. It is diagnosed with a blood test looking at the level of bile acids in the blood.

Vomiting in Pregnancy

It is normal to have some morning sickness in early pregnancy, however if a woman has severe vomiting, this is called hyperemesis gravidarum. This is when the pregnant woman is vomiting so much they are unable to stay hydrated. They are at high risk of malnutrition and dehydration and should be admitted to hospital for fluids and vitamin B1 (thiamine). The urine dip will show ketones.

In the second and third trimester, some women can still continue to experience morning sickness. However it is important to exclude pre-eclampsia and a urinary tract infection when assessing the patient.

> **Sita** was a 40 year old female who I met in my routine GP clinic. She was asked to see us by her community midwife. She was 1 week postpartum and had developed a mild headache. On further questioning, she felt a little 'puffy' in her feet. Her pregnancy was fairly unremarkable and she had delivered a baby boy by emergency cesarean section due to failure to progress. She had been kept in for one day and then discharged home. On examination her blood pressure was raised at 140/95. She had never been diagnosed with hypertension either before or during her pregnancy. Her urine dip showed 2+ of protein. I referred her back to the hospital

> where she was diagnosed with pre-eclampsia. This was a useful learning case which highlighted that pre-eclampsia can also occur in the post partum phase.

As in the previous chapters, I have created a list of presenting complaints in pregnancy. See if you can fill it in with the different differential diagnoses you should consider when taking the history.

Bleeding in early pregnancy	Bleeding in late pregnancy
Vomiting in pregnancy	Suprapubic pain in pregnancy
Itching in pregnancy	Headache in pregnancy

Answers

Bleeding in early pregnancy
– Miscarriage
– Ectopic pregnancy

Bleeding in late pregnancy
– Miscarriage
– Placental abruption

Vomiting in pregnancy
– Morning sickness
– Hyperemesis gravidarum
– Urinary tract infections
– Pre-elcampsia

Suprapubic pain in pregnancy
– Miscarriage
– Urinary tract infection

Itching in pregnancy
– PUPPS
– Pemphigoid gestationis
– Obstetric cholestasis

Headache in pregnancy
– Pre-eclampsia
– Usual causes of headache e.g. migraine, tension headache

Chapter 8. Obstetrics

Answer 6

This shows the common obstetric presenting complaints and possible differentials.

Practice Cases

Case 1

Instructions for the candidate:

> You are a GP. Your next patient is a 25 year old female. Please take a history and discuss your differential diagnoses.

Instructions for the actor:

> You are Emily Edwards, a 25 year old female who has come to her GP to discuss her periods.
>
> You have always had light periods but in the last 2 months it has become much more heavier and painful. You have also noticed some spotting between your periods. In the last 8 weeks you have also had a thick green discharge which is unusual for you.
>
> If asked, mention that sex is more painful. You have a deep pain in your lower abdomen during sex.
>
> If asked, mention that you have been in a new relationship for the last 3 months. You do not use condoms as you have the implant which you had inserted 1 year ago. Your last period was 10 days ago.
>
> Only if asked, mention that you had an STI check 6 months ago which was negative.
>
> PMH: You are fit and well. You had some asthma as a child but you don't need your inhaler anymore.
>
> NKDA
>
> FHX: nil of note

SHX: You work as a waitress and live with your sister. You have recently started dating a colleague at work.

ICE: You are worried about an STI and are feeling embarrassed by this. You would like some antibiotics for this.

Instructions for the examiner:

Criteria	Marks awarded
Elicits the presenting complaint (1)	
Asks the following – any unprotected sexual intercourse, any pain with sex, any bleeding with sex	
Asks about past medical history and family history (2)	
Asks about social history (1)	
Elicits ICE (1 mark)	
Total (max 10)	

The thick discharge and pelvic pain during intercourse suggest pelvic inflammatory disease. It is important that this patient is checked for STI's.

Case 2

Instructions for the candidate:

> You are a GP trainee doing the duty doctor clinic on a busy morning. Your next patient is a 70 year old female. Please take a history and discuss your differential diagnoses.

Instructions for the actor:

114 Chapter 8. Obstetrics

HPC: You are Mary Jones, a 70 year old retired pianist. You have come to see your GP because yesterday you noticed some blood in your underwear. You don't know why this happened and you are quite frightened. You do not have any stomach pain and there is no burning when you pass urine. Your bowels are ok. You have not seen any blood in your poo.

You reached the menopause 17 years ago. You suffered very badly with symptoms for the first few years but you were too scared to use HRT. You have not lost any weight but you have noticed your appetite is much less than it used to be.

PMH: You have hypertension and diabetes. Your diabetes is very mild and you take metformin once a day. You also take amlodipine.

No known drug allergies

Fhx: You don't remember if there is any family history of anything.

Shx: You are a retired pianist but you still enjoy playing the piano. You live with your husband who is retiring soon. You hope to go travelling together.

Instructions for the examiner:

Criteria	Marks awarded
Elicits the presenting complaint (1)	
Asks the following—any dysuria, problems with bowels, abdominal pain (3)	
Asks red flags—weight loss, loss of appetite (2)	
Asks about past medical history and family history (2)	

Asks about social history (1)

Elicits ICE (1 mark)

Total (max 10)

Any woman presenting with post menopausal bleeding needs to be assessed for endometrial cancer.

Case 3

Instructions for the candidate:

> You are an FY2 on your obstetrics and gynaecology rotation. You are covering the maternal foetal assessment unit. Your next patient is a 35 year old female who is 28 weeks pregnant. Please take a history and discuss your differential diagnoses.

Instructions for the actor:

> Your name is Emily Lee. You are 28 weeks pregnant with twins. This is your first pregnancy. The pregnancy has been going well, however over the last few weeks you have been feeling much more nauseous and started noticing your shoes are not fitting you properly. You thought this was normal in pregnancy but since yesterday you also have a severe headache which is not getting better. You used to get migraines when you were a teenager, but you have not had one in a long time.
>
> You do not have any bleeding or stomach pain. You have not vomited, but you do feel a little uncomfortable and nauseous. You have never been told that your blood pressure is high.
>
> You are fit and well. You do not have any medical problems. There is no family history of note.
>
> Social history – You live with your partner and you have a dog. You work as a financial advisor.
>
> You want to know if this is normal in pregnancy and you really need something strong to help with the headache as paracetamol is not enough.

Instructions for the examiner:

Criteria	Marks awarded
Elicits the presenting complaint (1)	
Asks the following—any abdominal pain, swelling of feet and hands, headache, vomiting (4)	
Asks about high blood pressure in pregnancy (1)	
Asks about past medical history and family history (2)	
Asks about social history (1)	
Elicits ICE (1 mark)	
Total (max 10)	

The history of raised blood pressure, headache and leg swelling is suggestive of preeclampsia. This patient will need blood tests, an up to date blood pressure and a urine dip.

Case 4

Instructions for the candidate:

> You are a GP trainee helping out the duty doctor. Your next patient is a 22 year old female with abdominal pain.

Instructions for the actor:

> You are Gina Dorris, a 22 year old student who has started having severe pain in her right lower abdomen. The pain woke you up this morning and you have been sick a few times. You don't have any PV bleeding and you do not have any diarrhoea. Only if asked, mention that you are slightly delayed with your period. You normally bleed every 30 days, but your last period was 6 weeks ago. You initially thought this was due to stress but you are now concerned you may be pregnant as you had some unprotected sex about 5 weeks ago when you were a little tipsy after a night out. You are too scared to do a pregnancy test as you are worried about

will happen if it is positive. You want to build a career for yourself and are not able to look after a baby right now.

PMH: You have asthma and take the brown inhaler regularly. You are allergic to penicillin.

There is no family history of note.

You are studying to be a dentist and are really enjoying your course. You are really worried that you may be pregnant and don't want your parents to find out.

Instructions for the examiner:

Criteria	Marks awarded
Elicits the presenting complaint (1)	
Asks the following—any vomiting, any bleeding, menstrual history, elicits chance of pregnancy (4)	
Asks about past medical history and family history (2)	
Asks about social history (1)	
Elicits ICE and in particular worries about family finding out (2 marks)	
Total (max 10)	

It is likely that this patient is pregnant. As she has unilateral pain she needs an urgent scan to rule out an ectopic pregnancy.

Case 5

Instructions for the candidate:

> You are an FY2 in general practice. Please take a history from Mrs. Emma Davis, a 60 year old female.

Instructions for the actor:

> You are Emma, a 60 year old retired teacher who has recently been feeling very bloated. You don't know what is triggering this, but you usually need to pop a

gaviscon after your meals. You don't have any pain, but you feel uncomfortable and gassy. You do not have any vomiting or diarrhoea but you are slightly constipated. You do not have any blood in your stool. You have started to eat less because of this discomfort, however your diet has not changed. You have not had any weight loss. Prior to this you have never had any problems with your gut. You have always had a healthy diet and taken care of yourself. This is rather unusual for you.

PMH: You have an underactive thyroid for which you take thyroxine. You recently had a blood test and was told your level is normal.

NKDA

Fhx: Your mother had breast cancer in her early 50's.

SHx: You are a retired teacher. You live with your husband and daughter. You are frustrated with these new symptoms and wonder if you may need something stronger to treat the indigestion.

Instructions for the examiner:

Criteria	Marks awarded
Elicits the presenting complaint (1)	
Asks the following—change in bowels, any vomiting, changes to diet (3)	
Asks red flags—PV bleeding/PR bleeding, weight loss/ loss of appetite (2)	
Asks about past medical history and family history (2)	
Asks about social history (1)	
Elicits ICE (1 marks)	
Total (max 10)	

Any new gut symptoms in an older woman should prompt you to think about ovarian cancer.

Chapter 9
Paediatric Histories

The Febrile Child

As a GP, I spend a lot of my day assessing children with fever. In the majority of cases, the cause is likely to be a viral illness, however we need to screen for any red flags and try and identify where the fever is coming from.

Causes of fever include:

Respiratory tract

Most of the time, the fever is likely to be related to a viral respiratory tract infection. The child may have a cough, runny nose, sore throat, ear pain and occasionally a blanching rash. When taking a history it is important to ask about any unwell contacts as well as any recent travel. Usually the fever responds to regular antipyretics and the child perks up between bouts of fever.

Common Viral Respiratory Tract Infections in Children

Sometimes we do not know exactly which virus is the cause of the illness. The child will have generic symptoms such as

TABLE 9.1 This shows common respiratory childhood viral infections

Condition	Symptoms
Bronchiolitis	Bronchiolitis is caused by the common cold virus (RSV). It occurs in young babies and children under the age of 2. As babies and toddlers have smaller airways, the infection can cause a mild wheeze and crackles. The nose is often blocked which can make it harder for them to feed (they rely more on mouth breathing when unwell and therefore are unable to feed for prolonged periods of time).
Viral induced wheeze	This is similar to bronchiolitis but occurs in slightly older children (6 months to 5 years). It is wheezing associated with infection. It is usually treated with a salbutamol inhaler to help them breathe more easily.
Croup	This is an infection of the upper airway caused by parainfluenza virus. It causes stridor (an inspiratory noise) due to inflammation of the upper airway. Children also have a barking cough. Often the child will need a single dose of steroids to help reduce the inflammation and make breathing easier.

sore throat, runny nose, ear pain and cough. A runny nose is a good indicator that the child has a viral illness. Bacterial infections are less likely to cause a runny nose. The following table describes three more specific viral illnesses in children (Table 9.1):

Occasionally, the infection may be a bacterial infection.

Bacterial Respiratory Tract Infections in Children (Table 9.2)

TABLE 9.2 This demonstrates bacterial infections which can occur in children

Lower respiratory tract infection	Children can also get bacterial pneumonia. This presents with a high fever. They may have a productive cough of yellow or green phlegm. On examination there may be crackles on auscultation.
Bacterial tonsillitis	Bacterial tonsillitis presents with enlarged painful and red tonsils. There may be white pus on the tonsils. Usually there is no cough or runny nose.
Scarlet fever	Scarlett fever is a condition which is linked to bacterial tonsillitis. The child also has systemic symptoms such as a sandpaper rash and strawberry tongue. It is caused by group A streptococcus.

Urinary Tract Infections

UTI's are slightly more common in young girls than boys. This is because the urethra is shorter in girls making it easier for bacteria to ascend upwards. If the child is verbal, they may complain of pain when passing urine. However if they are non-verbal, the only signs may be fever and vomiting. Therefore if the cause of the fever is unclear, it is important to try and get a urine sample from the child to check for a UTI.

If a child develops recurrent UTI's it may be important to refer them for a scan to look for any structural abnormalities in the renal tract.

Gastrointestinal

Children are also prone to getting gastroenteritis and may have diarrhoea and vomiting. It is important to assess the hydration status of the child. We will cover this in red flag questions.

Other Viral Infections (Table 9.3)

Rarer Causes of Fever in a Child (Table 9.4)

Questions to ask when assessing a child with fever:

- The first step is trying to identify the source of the fever, which we have just discussed.
- Following this, it is important to determine how sick the child is. The following information is important to ask:
  - Are they drinking enough fluids? — it is important that the child stays hydrated. When a child is sick, parents often worry that they are not eating enough. Food intake is not as important as fluid intake. If the child is vomiting and unable to keep fluids down, this is an indication for them to go to hospital.
  - Are they passing enough urine? — Another indication that a child is hydrated is if they are passing enough

TABLE 9.3 This shows other childhood viral infections

Chicken pox	This is a viral illness caused by varicella zoster. It causes a prodrome of fever and malaise. The rash is a blistering rash all over the body. It is extremely itchy and very contagious.
Hand foot and mouth	This is caused by an enterovirus. It presents with fever and a blistering rash typically on the palms, soles and inside of the mouth. It is a self limiting condition.
Fifths disease	This is also known as 'slapped cheek syndrome' and is caused by parvovirus. The children may present with fever and a runny nose. They usually have a bright red rash on one or both cheeks which is where the name comes from.
Sixths disease	This is also known as Roseola Infantum. It is caused by the human herpes virus type 6. It presents with a high fever. Once this resolves, a rash usually appears all over the body.

TABLE 9.4 This table shows rare causes of fever in children

Osteomyelitis	This is an infection of the bone. See the section on the limping child.
Meningitis	This is an infection of the meninges which cover the brain. Children may complain of a headache and photophobia. They will have neck stiffness and a high fever. If the cause is *Nisseria meningitidis*, they will develop a non-blanching rash over their body. Meningitis is a medical emergency.
Kawasaki disease	This is a vasculitis rather than an infection, however it presents with a prolonged temperature (more than 5 days). Other symptoms include: – Dry lips – Strawberry tongue – Swollen feet – Enlarged lymph nodes – Conjunctivitis – Rash It is important to diagnose this as there may be cardiac involvement. Always consider Kawasaki disease in a child with a fever for more than 5–10 days without a clear source.
Fever of unknown origin	Sometimes, we are not able to find out where the fever is coming from. It is always important to check for any recent travel to exclude the possibility of a tropical disease like malaria. Malignancy can also cause fever of unknown origin.

urine. In a baby or younger child, you can ask if they are producing the same number of wet nappies as normal. If they are producing less than 50% of the normal amount of nappies then this suggests that they are dehydrated or hemodynamically unstable and need to go to hospital.

- Do they have any rashes? In particular any child with a non-blanching rash needs to go straight to hospital due to concerns about meningitis.
- Are they up to date with their immunisations? — an unimmunised child is at a higher risk of rare causes of fever such as measles.
- Any recent travel? It is important to keep in mind tropical diseases such as malaria.
- A really good resource to familiarise yourself with is the traffic light system. This was designed to give us an idea about how sick a child is and when to refer them to hospital.

Enuresis — Bed Wetting

It is normal for children to wet the bed up to a certain age — usually around 5 years of age. However in some cases, older children may continue to wet the bed. The term for this is enuresis and there are two types:

1. Primary enuresis - this is bed wetting in a child older than the age of 5 who has never achieved night time dryness. There are two main subtypes which depend on whether the child has daytime symptoms or not. In a child without any daytime symptoms, the main management is reassuring parents and providing advice about conservative ways to help the child achieve night time continence. In a child with daytime symptoms, it is important to exclude a UTI and constipation. Once this has been done, it would be sensible to refer them to secondary care to consider other causes e.g. neurological causes.
2. Secondary enuresis — this is bed wetting in a child that has previously been dry for 6 months.

When taking a secondary enuresis history, it is important to consider the following differential diagnoses (Table 9.5):

TABLE 9.5 This table shows the possible causes of bedwetting which must be considered during the history

Cause	Other symptoms
UTI	If the child has a UTI, this may lead to urinary frequency and bed wetting
Type 1 diabetes	Type 1 diabetes can present with urinary frequency and excessive thirst. It can also present with weight loss and failure to thrive
Constipation	Constipation can cause the bowels to stretch and press on the bladder. This can make it harder to control bladder function.
Psychological	The commonest cause of secondary enuresis in children is psychological. A stressful life event or big change e.g. moving house/ school can manifest as secondary nocturnal enuresis. Therefore it is important to take a good social history.
Neurological	This is rare but should be considered if the child has persistent daytime symptoms.

Abdominal Pain

The causes of abdominal pain in children is similar to the causes of abdominal pain in adults. However some conditions are more common than others.

Acute Abdominal Pain

1. Children can get appendicitis, and this presents in the same way as adults.
2. Gastroenteritis—fever, diarrhoea and vomiting
3. Mesenteric adenitis—This is inflammation of the glands that lie inside the abdomen. They become inflamed in response to a viral or bacterial infection. Therefore consider mesenteric adenitis if the child has had a recent viral illness or upper respiratory tract infection.

126 Chapter 9. Paediatric Histories

4. Testicular torsion—this is when the testes twists on its axis. It can cause pain and swelling of the scrotum as well as abdominal pain. In any young boy with unexplained abdominal pain, it is important to check the scrotum. This is a surgical emergency due to the risk of avascular necrosis of the testes.
5. Urinary tract infections
6. Intussusception—This is a condition in which the bowel telescopes in on itself (Figure 9.1). This can lead to loss of

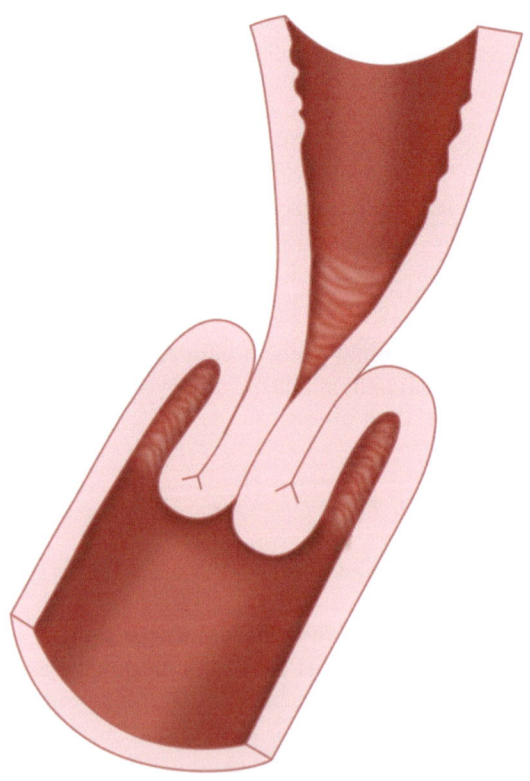

Figure 9.1 This diagram shows the bowel telescoping in on itself in intussusception

blood supply to the bowel. It usually presents between the age of 3–18 months. Symptoms include abdominal pain, fever and blood in the stool. The child may be irritable and will often draw their knees to their chest.
7. Diabetic ketoacidosis (DKA) — Sometimes kids with type 1 diabetes may be undiagnosed and present with DKA. The symptoms of this include weight loss, increased thirst, increased urinary frequency, abdominal pain and nausea and sometimes vomiting. The breath may smell sweet because of the ketones. There may be a family history of autoimmune disease.

Chronic Abdominal Pain

1. The commonest cause of chronic abdominal pain in children is constipation. It's important to ask for a detailed bowel history and dietary history. A useful tip is to bring up the Bristol stool chart and ask the child to point to what their 'poo' looks like. Although constipation is usually due to lifestyle or behaviour, you need to consider other causes like an underactive thyroid or Hirschsprung's disease. This is a neurological condition due to the absence of nerves at the distal end of the bowel which means that peristalsis cannot occur normally. It is usually diagnosed at birth as the child fails to pass meconium. However, in some cases, diagnosis can be delayed.
2. Some children also hold their bowels when they are in school which can cause discomfort and faecal impaction over time. They may even develop overflow diarrhoea from the impaction. It is important to enquire about toileting habits in children.
3. Other rare causes include coeliac disease and inflammatory bowel disease. If there is a strong family history of autoimmune disease or if there is failure to thrive (see below) then it is important to test for these conditions in any child with abdominal pain or abnormal bowels.

> **Mindy** was a 5 year old girl who was booked in to see the GP by her mother. She had been suffering with constipation for many years and had now developed an anal fissure which made it very painful to open her bowels. On further questioning, it transpired that she had some vitiligo and there was a very strong family history of autoimmune disease. Blood tests were arranged and she was subsequently diagnosed with coeliac disease.

Failure to Thrive

When a baby is born, their weight is regularly plotted on to a chart to make sure that the weight is increasing steadily. If a child's weight starts to drop this is called failure to thrive. Causes of failure to thrive can be divided into the following categories. Table 9.6 is not comprehensive but gives you an idea of how to think about the different causes of failure to thrive:

TABLE 9.6 This shows the possible cause of failure to thrive

Pathology	causes	questions to ask
Reduced intake of food	– Child abuse – Poverty – Feeding difficulties e.g. tongue tie, developmental problems which affect feeding – Severe reflux – Pyloric stenosis	– Food intake – Swallowing difficulties – Vomiting
Reduced absorption of food	Coeliac disease Inflammatory bowel disease Cystic fibrosis Food allergies	– Abdominal pain – Bowel habits – Family history of autoimmune disease or allergies
Increased use of energy	Cancer Hyperthyroidism	– Symptoms of hyperthyroidism or malignancy

Developmental Disorders

This is a very wide topic, however we will focus on two key areas—motor delay and speech delay.

Motor Delay

Common causes of this include.

1. Cerebral palsy—This is a condition caused by brain damage during pregnancy or delivery. It can present with learning difficulties as well as muscle spasticity.
2. Autism spectrum disorder—This is a spectrum of behavioural abnormalities in children. These behavioural abnormalities are usually related to

    (a) problems with social communication e.g. difficulty with speech
    (b) repetitive behaviours. They may also have some problems with gross and fine motor skills.
    (c) problems with social interaction e.g. playing with other children, problems with eye contact

3. Genetic conditions

    – Downs syndrome—this is due to trisomy 21. It causes learning difficulties as well as problems with motor development. The child may have physical features of Downs syndrome. These include (Table 9.7)

Table 9.7 Features that may be seen in an individual with Down's syndrome

Flattened face
Single palmar crease
Webbed feet
Protruding tongue
Short stature

- Inherited neuromuscular conditions — The main group of conditions are the muscular dystrophies. Duchenne muscular dystrophy presents with delayed walking in children. Often the children will be wheelchair bound before they are teenagers.

Speech and Language Delay

1. Hearing impairment — children with hearing impairment will also have delayed speech. This is because hearing is key to normal speech development. A common cause of hearing loss in children is glue ear or chronic otitis media. It is therefore important to ask about a history of ear infections in the child.
2. Learning multiple languages at once — children who are exposed to multiple languages at the same time can sometimes begin to speak slightly later, however this is temporary and should still be within the normal range of language development.
3. Down's syndrome — It is not uncommon for children with Down's syndrome to have speech delay.
4. Autism spectrum disorder — Autism spectrum disorder may present with speech delay and difficulties with social interaction.
5. Fragile X syndrome — This is a genetic disorder which can cause developmental problems. Individuals will typically have a phenotype which includes large ears, long face and a high arched palate. They often have speech and language delays.
6. Speech dyspraxia — This is a problem with the articulation and pronunciation of words. The lack of coordination of muscles in the oral cavity and pharynx can sometimes cause problems with eating and swallowing.
7. Physical abnormalities such as a cleft palate can make speaking difficult.

Rashes in Children

Rashes are a common presenting complaint in children. You can divide rashes up into acute and chronic.

The following table is a useful guide to deciphering the cause of a rash in a child. The list is comprehensive but not exhaustive.

Acute Rashes (Table 9.8)

Chronic Rashes

Common chronic rashes in children include:

1. eczema—eczema is a condition which causes dry skin. It is often found in the following areas:
   infants: face, scalp.
   babies and toddlers: elbows, knees
2. Psoriasis—this is an autoimmune skin condition which causes scaly plaques to form on the body. Unlike eczema which tends to form on the flexural surface of the elbow and knees (back of the knee and front of the elbow), psoriasis is found on the extensor surface (front of the knee and back of the elbow).
3. Mollucscum contagiosum—this is a viral condition which causes asymptomatic umbilicated papules to form around the body. The lesions are very contagious and can take months to clear.

TABLE 9.8 This table goes through the different types of childhood rashes as well as the possible causes

Type of rash	Causes	Symptoms
Maculopapular	In children the commonest cause of this would be a viral infection. The rash is typically blanching and accompanies a fever, sore throat and cough.	Blanching rash, Not itchy All over the body Accompanied by other infective symptoms
Vesicular	Chicken pox	This presents with a widespread itchy vesicular rash all over the body. It is accompanied by fever.
	Shingles	This is a similar rash to chickenpox but it only presents in one dermatome. It is caused by reactivation of the chicken pox virus.
	Hand foot and mouth	This can also lead to the development of vesicles in the hands, feet and inside of the mouth.

(continued)

TABLE 9.8 (continued)

Type of rash	Causes	Symptoms
Petechial	Meningococcal meningitis	This presents with fever, headache, neck stiffness and a non-blanching rash. It is a medical emergency.
	Idiopathic thrombocytopenia	This is an autoimmune condition which causes platelets to get destroyed. The low platelets leads to easy bruising and petechia appearing over the body.
	Henoch Scholein purpura	This is a form of vasculitis which affects the kidneys, joints and skin. It presents with a purpuic rash on the buttock and back of the legs. The children may also have haematuria.

The Limping Child

If a child has a limp with fever, you should consider the following:

With Fever

1. Septic arthritis/ osteomyelitis—This is infection of the joint or bone. The child will have a fever. The joint may be red, hot and swollen. Often the child is unable to move the joint due to the severity of the pain and inflammation.
2. Transient synovitis—This is inflammation of the hip following a viral illness. It usually self resolves.

It is very important to exclude septic arthritis in any child with a fever and limp.

Without Fever

1. Injury — accidental and non-accidental
2. Juvenile arthritis — This is an autoimmune condition which causes joint pains and swelling in children under the age of 16 years of age. It is similar to rheumatoid arthritis in adults.
3. Slipped upper femoral epiphysis — This usually occurs between the ages of 11–17. It is caused by the femoral head slipping backwards in the joint. It presents with pain in the hip, a limp and restricted movements.
4. Perthes disease — This is caused by disruption of the blood supply to the hip bone. This causes necrosis of the bone. It presents with pain, a limp and restricted movement. Most children recover without any treatment. It usually occurs between the ages of 4–10.
5. Developmental dysplasia of the hip — This is a condition which is usually diagnosed at birth but may be missed. It is due to abnormal formation of the hip joint which leads to the hip joint being more easily to dislocate. It can lead to differences in leg length, limping and waddling.

Questions to Ask in a Child with a Limp

1. Any fever - if they have a fever they need to be assessed urgently to exclude septic arthritis.
2. Any injury? — if they have had an injury you need to consider a fracture. You also need to keep in mind the possibility of child abuse.
3. Any other joint involvement or any rash? This may suggest an autoimmune cause
4. How long has the problem been going on for? Is it triggered by sport or exercise?

As I did in the previous chapter, I have created some tables for you to fill in to help you understand the differential diagnosis for common presenting complaints.

Rashes in Children

Fever and cough	Fever and a rash
Acute abdominal pain	Chronic abdominal pain
Fever and limp	Limp without a fever
Vomiting	Diarrhoea
Bed wetting	

Answers

Fever and cough	Fever and a rash
Viral respiratory tract infection	5th's disease
Croup	6th's disease
Bronchiolitis	Chicken pox
Bacterial respiratory tract infection	Hand foot and mouth
	Scarlett fever

Acute abdominal pain	Chronic abdominal pain
Appendicitis	Constipation
Gastroenteritis	IBD
Intussusception	Coeliac disease
DKA	

Fever and limp	Limp without a fever
Osteomyelitis/ septic arthritis	Perthes disease
Transient synovitis	Injury—Accidental/ non-accidental
	Slipped upper femoral epiphysis
	Developmental dysplasia of the hip

Vomiting	Diarrhoea
Gastroenteritis	Gastroenteritis
Pyloric stenosis	Coeliac disease
DKA	Overflow diarrhoea from constipation
Urinary tract infection	
(rare cause – brain tumour)	Inflammatory bowel disease
	Intussusception

Bed wetting
Psychological
UTI
Diabetes
Neurological causes

Answers 7

This shows the common paediatric presenting complaints and possible differentials.

Paediatric Cases to Practise

Case 1

Instructions for the candidate:

> You are a GP trainee doing your morning clinic. Your next patient is Freddie, a 10 year old boy who has come to see you with his mum. Please take a history and discuss your differential diagnosis.

Instructions for the actor:

> HPC: You are the mum of Freddie, a well 10 year old boy.
> You are worried as he has started wetting the bed recently. It was initially once in a while and now it is

almost every day. He stopped wetting the bed at the age of 6, but this has started all of a sudden.

There are no concerns with him leaking in the day and it does not hurt when he passes water. He is upset by the bed wetting as it embarasses him and he is worried about an upcoming overnight school trip. He is gaining weight and is otherwise well. He is not more thirsty than normal and usually doesn't drink much in the evening.

PMH: Nil. He was born at term and has had no problems with development. He takes some vitamins and does not have any allergies.

FHX: There is no family history of note.

Shx: He lives with you and your husband. You are in the process of separating from your husband and both of you will co-parent Freddie. You also have a 6 year old daughter.

ICE: You are worried about the impact this is having on his confidence and also his sleep and would like to get to the bottom of this.

Instructions for the examiner:

Elicits the presenting complaint (1)
Elicits the following—if previously dry, no daytime symptoms, any dysuria, polyuria, upcoming school trip (5)
Asks about past medical history and family history (2)
Asks about social history and in particular the problems in the marriage (1)
asks about ICE (1)
Total (10)

Freddie is suffering from secondary enuresis. The lack of daytime symptoms is reassuring. It is important to check his urine for infection and glucose, however it is likely that the cause of this is psychological given that his parents are separating.

Chapter 9. Paediatric Histories

Case 2

Instructions for the candidate:

> You are an FY2 doing a paediatrics rotation. Your next patient in A + E is a 6 month old baby with a cough and fever. Please take a history and discuss your differential diagnosis.

Instructions for the actor:

> You are the mum of Samantha, a 6 month old baby girl. She developed a fever yesterday night. She is coughing and she sounds like she has a blocked nose. Only if asked, mention that your husband thought she sounded like a dog when she coughed. You have also noticed that when she is upset she makes a funny noise in her throat. This settles down when she is happier. You have not travelled anywhere recently, but she does go to nursery 1 day a week so may have picked up something from there. She is breast and bottle fed although she is drinking much less than usual. She is still passing aout 60–70% of her normal wet nappies. She does not have a rash on her body.
>
> PMH: She was born at 38 weeks gestation via a forceps delivery. She has been well since and is up to date with her vaccinations.
>
> Fhx: You have asthma and nut allergies.
>
> Shx: Samantha lives with you and your partner. You do not have any more children.
>
> ICE: You are really worried about the cough and think she may need antibiotics.

Instructions for the examiner:

Elicits the presenting complaint (1)

Elicits the following -fever, rash, oral intake & urine output, nature of the cough (4)

Asks about past medical history, immunisation history and family history (3)

Asks about social history (1)

asks about ICE (1)

Total (10)

The barking cough makes a diagnosis of croup very likely. Croup is treated with a small dose of dexamethasone to help relax the upper airway and improve their breathing. It is important to ask about oral intake and hydration status in any child with a fever.

Case 3

Instructions for the candidate:

> You are a GP doing your morning clinic. Your next patient is Ralph, a 15 year old boy. Please take a history and discuss your differential diagnoses.

Instructions for the actor:

> You are Ralph, a 15 year old boy. You have been experiencing pain in your left hip and groin for the last 2 weeks. This is worse when you walk and you are unable to play football anymore. Your mum mentioned that you have now started limping.
>
> You have not injured yourself and are normally very sporty. There is no joint swelling or redness and you do not have a fever. If asked, mention that you have always been slightly overweight.
>
> You have eczema which is controlled with moisturisers and steroid creams.
>
> You are allergic to nuts and penicillin.
>
> Fhx: Your grandfather has arthritis. You don't know much about this, but he did have an operation of this 2 years ago.
>
> Shx: You go to school and love playing football. You are worried you will never be able to play again. You have an important tournament next month and want to play. You live with your parents and older sister.

Instructions for the examiner:

Elicits the presenting complaint (1)
Elicits the following -fever, limp, injury, swelling (4)
Asks about past medical history, and family history (2)
Asks about social history and about concerns re football (2)
asks about ICE (1)
Total (10)

The most likely diagnosis is slipped upper femoral epiphysis. It occurs in adolescents and risk factors include being overweight or having a family history.

Case 4

Instructions for the candidate:

> You are an FY2 doctor doing a night shift in paediatric A + E. Your next patient is Miles, an 8 year old boy. He has come to see you with his mother, Elena. Please take a history and discuss your differential diagnosis.

Instructions for the actor:

> You are the mum of Miles. He is 8 years old and over the last few months you have felt that something is not quite right. He has been losing weight drinking a lot of juice and water. However over the last 2 days he has been complaining of central stomach pain. He has vomited a few times earlier today which is why you brought him in. There is no blood in the vomit, it is a whitish/green colour. He does not have a fever, but he looks very unwell. He last opened his bowels 2 days ago, it was normal. He is passing urine much more frequently but is not complaining it's hurting. Only if asked, mention that you noticed his breath smells quite sweet.

PMH: He is fit and well. He has been under the weather recently with a viral illness, however this has now settled.

He has no allergies

Fhx: You have Graves disease which was treated with carbimazole.

Shx: You are a single mum following your divorce 2 years ago. Your partner helps co-parent Miles.

Instructions for the examiner:

Elicits the presenting complaint (1)

Asks the following -polyuria, polydipsia, vomiting, sweet smelling breath, fever (5)

Asks about past medical history, and family history (2)

Asks about social history (1)

Asks about ICE (1)

Total (10)

The vague abdominal pain, vomiting and weight loss all point towards a possible diagnosis of diabetic ketoacidosis. It is important to check the capillary glucose or perform a urine dip to assess for glucose and ketones.

Case 5

You are working in the urgent care centre. Your next patient is a 5 year old boy, Tim. He has come to see you with his father. Please take a history and discuss your differential diagnosis.

Instructions for the actor:

You are the dad of Tim. You have brought him in as you have noted that he has a red bruise like rash on the back of his legs. The rash does not disappear when you put pressure on it. This came on quite quickly. He has been complaining of feeling generally unwell for a few weeks with occasional headaches and leg pain. You thought the leg pains were growing pains at the time which is why you didn't take him to the doctor. You have not noticed any joint swelling. He has also had some vague abdominal pain and has also been off his food recently. There is no fever, photophobia and he does not have any neck stiffness.

PMH: He was born at 34 weeks as his mother went into premature labour. He was in NICU for a few days but since coming home has been fine. He has no past medical history.

He has no allergies

Fhx: nil of note

Shx: He lives with you and your partner. She was not able to come today as she is in her third trimester of pregnancy.

Instructions for the examiner:

Elicits the presenting complaint (1)

Asks the following -abdominal pain, fever, if the rash is blanching, joint pain, headache (5)

Asks about past medical history, and family history (2)

Asks about social history (1)

asks about ICE (1)

Total (10)

The description of the rash is suggestive of a petechial rash. It is likely to be Henloch Scholein Purpura given the distribution of the rash. The next investigation would be a blood test to assess platelet count, kidney function and inflammatory markers as well as a urine dip. The blood pressure will also need to be checked as renal involvement can cause a high blood pressure.

Chapter 10
Psychiatry

Low Mood

If a patient presents with low mood, they may have depression. Depression can be classified into mild, moderate and severe. The patient may complain of psychical and psychological symptoms (Table 10.1):

When assessing someone with depression, as mentioned earlier, the main concern is ensuring they are safe. Assessing for suicidal risk is extremely important.

Other important questions to ask include the 4 W's:

- **Why?** has anything triggered the depression? has there been a major life event? There is often an overlap between grief and depression. It is normal to feel sad and have a low mood for a few months after a bereavement. However grief normally improves over time and the feelings are focused on the loss of a loved one. On the other hand, depression may not improve and the symptoms include worthlessness and low self esteem which are not linked to the loss.
- **When?** How long have they been feeling like this? have they had depression/low mood in the past or is this a new symptom.
- **Who?** Who do they have to support them? Do they have family close by, are they living with anyone? In

TABLE 10.1 This table shows both the physical and psychological symptoms of depression

Physical symptoms	Psychological
Unable to sleep/excessive sleep	Low mood
Unable to eat/binge eating	Feeling angry or guilty
Loss of interest in doing things they previously used to do	Tearful
Social isolation	Negative thought pattern
Lack of concentration	
Fatigue	
Memory loss	

someone with severe depression, it is also important to assess if there are any children living with them as there may be a safeguarding element.
- **What?** Some people try to numb their symptoms through the use of drugs and alcohol and sometimes the drug/ alcohol use leads to depression. Therefore it is important to take a detailed drug history.
- It is also important to enquire if they have been or are on any medication for depression such as selective serotonin reuptake inhibitors (SSRI's).

It is also important to assess for symptoms of mania alongside depression, to ensure the patient does not have Bipolar disorder.

Bipolar disorder is a condition in which an individual fluctuates between depression and mania. In the manic phase they may have delusions (inaccurate beliefs), they often speak fast, are unable to sleep much and they take part in risky behaviours.

There may be an overlap with low mood and other conditions such as anxiety and PTSD (see below).

Anxiety/Worry

There is an overlap between depression and anxiety and often patients present with both. Anxiety is a condition in which a patient worries a lot. There are many different types of anxiety disorders and sometimes they overlap. The common ones include:

1. Generalised anxiety disorder—this is when a patient worries about a range of different things. It can have a huge impact on their daily life.
2. Panic disorder—In this condition patients develop panic attacks. They suddenly start to feel chest pain, shortness of breath, tingling in their hands. They often think that they are going to die. It can be very frightening for them.
3. Obsessive compulsive disorder—in this condition, patients have unpleasant obsessive thoughts which are uncomfortable and anxiety provoking. They subsequently develop compulsive and ritualistic behaviours to help ease this anxiety. Such behaviours include compulsive hand washing, checking doors and switches repeatedly, praying.

In patients who present with depression + − anxiety, it is important to consider other systemic causes of this. These include thyroid abnormalities and electrolyte abnormalities. Therefore it may be appropriate to arrange a blood test (Table 10.2):

TABLE 10.2 This table shows organic causes of fatigue, low mood and anxiety which should be excluded in a patient with depression and/or anxiety

TSH	Hypothyroidism may lead to depression and hyperthyroidism can present with anxiety
Hb/ iron	Anaemia can cause fatigue and tiredness
Calcium	High calcium levels can affect your mood
Vitamin D	Low vitamin D can also cause fatigue and body pain.

> When I was a GP trainee, I met Alison, a 24 year old female with severe anxiety. She was already on an antidepressant, however her symptoms continued to have a big impact on her life.
>
> Following a consultation with her, I decided to do a routine blood test. To my surprise, her thyroid function was deranged. She was diagnosed with hyperthyroidism and referred to endocrinology. Once her TSH and T4 were in the normal range, her anxiety symptoms dramatically improved. Therefore it is always important to keep in mind organic causes of anxiety and depression.

Hallucinations

A Hallucination is when a person experiences something that is not really there.

Common forms of hallucinations include:

>auditory hallucinations: hearing voices that do not exist
>visual hallucinations: seeing visuals (e.g. people, animals) that are not there.

There are many causes of hallucinations (Table 10.3).

You may hear the word psychosis being used in psychiatry. Hallucinations are just one symptom of psychosis. This is defined as an impairment in mental state that results in an individual losing touch with reality. If a person is psychotic, they may have

- hallucinations
- delusions
- Abnormal thoughts

The commonest causes of psychosis include schizophrenia, bipolar disease and drug induced psychosis. Damage to the brain such as infections and malignancy can also cause someone to become psychotic.

It is time for you to practise grouping your differential diagnoses together based on the presenting complaints.

TABLE 10.3 This table shows the organic and non-organic causes of hallucinations

Drug/alcohol withdrawal	Delirium tremens is a symptom of alcohol withdrawal. One of the ways it presents is with tactile hallucinations. The patient may feel that bugs are crawling over his or her skin.
Schizophrenia	This is a mental health condition which presents with hallucinations and delusions. Delusions are when a person has false beliefs that they believe they are true. For example they may have a fixed belief that they are the queen.
Bipolar disorder	Alongside low mood, patients with bipolar disorder also experience symptoms of mania, of which hallucinations is one of them. They may also experience delusions.
Lewy Body Dementia	We discussed Lewy body dementia earlier on in the chapter on confusion. It is a form of dementia which can present with hallucinations. Typically they will see people or animals (but not always).
Post traumatic stress disorder	PTSD is a condition caused by a distressing event. Following this they have low mood, irritability, and flashbacks. They may also have visual hallucinations as a result of the flashback.
Drug use	Many drugs cause patients to experience hallucinations. These include prescription and non-prescription drugs. For example, the painkiller tramadol can cause some individuals to experience hallucinations.
Severe depression	Sometimes, someone who is severely depressed may hear auditory hallucinations which are derogatory in nature.
Brain tumours	Depending on where it is, a brain tumour can cause hallucinations.

Low mood	Anxiety
Hallucinations	Delusions

Answers

Low mood	Anxiety
Depression	Thyrotoxicosis
Anxiety	Generalised anxiety disorders
Bipolar disorder	Phobias
Bereavement	Panic disorder
Anaemia	OCD
Low vitamin D	
Hypercalcaemia	

Hallucinations	Delusions
Drugs	Bipolar disorder
Dementia	Schizophrenia
Bipolar disorder	Drug use
Schizophrenia	Severe depression
PTSD	Brain injury e.g. cancer or infection

Answer 8

This shows the common psychiatric presenting complaints and possible differentials.

Cases to Practise

Case 1

Instructions for the candidate:

> You are a GP doing your afternoon clinic. Your next patient is Jaqueline, a 35 year old female. Please take a history and discuss your differential diagnosis.

Cases to Practise   149

Instructions for the candidate:

> You are Jaqueline, a 35 year old investment banker who has been feeling rather low for the last few months. This is getting worse and you feel you are at crisis point.
>
> This also started when you went through a breakdown of your marriage. You are prone to low mood and have had bouts of depression in the past. Since the divorce you have lost interest in doing anything. You don't eat much, but occasionally you binge eat and then purge. You stopped talking to your friends, as a lot of your friends were mutual friends and you used to spend time together as a couple. You sleep too much, but still feel exhausted when you wake up. You have to force yourself to go to work.
>
> If asked, mention that you have started drinking regularly and have a couple of glasses of wine every night. You have had suicidal thoughts, but will not act on these at the moment as you are very close to your parents. They have been very supportive and they have suggested you move back in with them. You are considering whether this may be a good idea in the short term.
>
> PMH: You have seborrheic dermatitis for which you use a special shampoo. You do not have any allergies.
>
> Fhx: Your dad suffered from depression in his twenties and thirties. He was on antidepressants for many years.
>
> Shx: You live alone in a rented flat. You don't smoke and do not take any other recreational drugs. You don't have any children.
>
> ICE: You think you may need antidepressants and would like to get a prescription for this.

Instructions for the examiner:

Elicits the presenting complaint (1)

Asks the following—recent life event, suicidal thoughts, eating and sleeping (4)

Asks about past medical history, and family history (2)

Asks about social history including drugs/ alcohol and if she has any children (2) asks about ICE (1)

Total (10)

This history is suggestive of someone who has depression. It is important to assess for suicide risk. In this case, the patient is not at immediate risk of suicide but does need to be closely monitored. You can start her on antidepressants, however be aware that in the first week after starting the medication, patients may feel worse and need to be followed up regularly.

Case 2

Instructions for the examiner:

> You are an FY2 in A + E. Your next patient has been brought in by the police. He has been found by the police looking slightly confused. Please take a history and discuss your differential diagnosis.

Instructions for the actor:

> Your name is Jeremy Brown and you are a 28 year old man. You have been brought in by the police. They didn't believe you when you told them that there was a man chasing you with a knife. They said they could not see anyone. If asked if you feel unwell, mention that you are a little shaky and sweaty. You are craving a drink as you can't remember when you last had a pint.
>
> You have also been feeling very itchy. You think your clothes have been contaminated with bugs. You have been scratching like crazy. If asked, mention you vomited a little bit earlier.
>
> PMH: you don't have any medical conditions that you know of, but you haven't seen your doctor in many years
>
> FHX: nil—you don't speak to your family.
>
> Shx—You are currently homeless and live in a homeless shelter when you get space.

You drink a few pints a day when you have money. You last drank 2–3 days ago because you don't have any money at the moment.

You don't take any drugs now, but you have done some heroin in the past.

ICE: You think the police are not treating you fairly. You feel that your life is in danger from the armed man. You can still see him and want someone to help you.

Instructions for the examiner:

Elicits the presenting complaint (1)

Asks the following — tremors, sweating, hallucinations, vomiting (4)

Asks about past medical history, and family history (2)

Asks about social history including alcohol and drug use. Extra point for eliciting homelessness (2)

asks about ICE (1)

Total (10)

These symptoms are suggestive of someone who is likely to be in delirium tremens due to alcohol withdrawal.

Case 3

Instructions for the candidate:

> You are a GP doing a routine clinic. Your next patient is Emma, an 18 year old female. Please take a history and discuss your differentials.

Instructions for the actor:

> You are Emma, an 18 year old student who has been suffering with worrying thoughts. You have been too embarrassed to speak to anyone about this but it is now impacting your life. You keep worrying that you are going to fall sick and therefore have to wash your hands

every 30–60 min to feel relief. Your hands are cracked and very dry.

You also worry a lot about house fires and have to check all of the plugs before you leave the house.

These symptoms are really affecting your confidence and you are feeling very isolated as you are embarrassed to share this with anyone.

Your mood is okay, although the anxiety can be debilitating at times. You are sleeping ok and eat well. You do not have any thoughts to hurt yourself.

PMH: You don't have any medical problems.

Drug hx—nil and no known allergies

Fhx—you have a family history of high blood pressure and breast cancer.

Shx—You have just started university and are struggling to make friends due to your anxiety. This is really frustrating and you really want to have this problem sorted out. You are still able to study, but constantly use sanitisers every hour which people find weird.

ICE—You read somewhere about prozac being used for anxiety and would like a prescription for this. You hope it will start to work immediately.

Instructions for the examiner:

Elicits the presenting complaint (1)

Asks the following—low mood, compulsions, suicidal ideation, eating/ sleeping (4)

Asks about past medical history, and family history (2)

Asks about social history including the effect of symptoms on ability to function. (2)

Asks about ICE (1)

Total (10)

The likely diagnosis here is OCD. The patient is complaining of obsessive thoughts and compulsions which help relieve her anxiety. The treatment would involve cognitive behavioural therapy (CBT) and/or SSRI's.

Case 4

Instructions for the candidate:

> You are a GP trainee. Your next patient is the mother of a 21 year old man. Please take a history and discuss your differential diagnosis.

Instructions for the actor:

> You are Genelia, the mother of Jerome. He is 21 years old. You came to the doctor today as you are really worried about his behaviour. Over the last few months he has become withdrawn and barely speaks to anyone. He stays alone in his room. You sometimes hear him talking out loud, telling someone to leave him alone. You don't know who he is talking to. You have also noticed that he doesn't eat anymore. He keeps saying that Dave has poisoned his food. You don't know if Dave is someone he knows.
>
> He normally works at the local supermarket but hasn't been going to work for the last week. You are really worried about his health. You have never seen him carry a gun or knife and he has never expressed any suicidal thoughts.
>
> PMH: He has thalassaemia trait.
>
> No known allergies
>
> Fhx: There is no family history of note. If asked about any mental health history in the family, mention that your mother has schizophrenia.
>
> Shx: If asked regarding drugs and alcohol, mention that you don't know what he gets up to in his spare time. He occasionally smokes weed because you can smell it in the house.
>
> You live alone with him. His father has never been part of your family.

ICE: You are really concerned about your son. You want to know if he has been to the doctor recently and what might be going on.

Instructions for the examiner:

Elicits the presenting complaint (1)

Asks the following – possible hallucinations, delusions, withdrawn behaviour, suicidal ideation 4)

Asks about past medical history, and family history (2)

Asks about living situation and drug use (2)

asks about ICE (1)

Total (10)

This case is likely a new diagnosis of schizophrenia. Often individuals become withdrawn and they have hallucinations and delusions.

Case 5

Instructions for the candidate:

> You are working in a GP practice. Your next patient is a 27 year old female. Please take a history and discuss your differential diagnoses.

Instructions for the actor:

> Your name is Amelia and you are 27 years old. You have recently noticed some strange symptoms which come on everytime you go onto public transport. You feel your chest become tight and you struggle to breathe. It is a horrible sensation and it makes you panic. It normally settles after some deep breathing.
> If asked, mention you also get palpitations as well as tingling in your hands and feet. You never used to get this, however since the pandemic began you have noticed these symptoms.
> You are fine the rest of the time.

You do have a history of mild anxiety for which you have had some cognitive behavioural therapy. You have been more stressed at work recently, but apart from this, nothing else has changed. You have felt overwhelmed about going back to working in the office after working from home for the last 18 months.
PMH: acne for which you use benzoyl peroxide cream.
Medications—the oral contraceptive pill.
You have an allergy to latex.
Fhx: high cholesterol and heart disease.
Shx: You work in a bank. You have to go in 3 times a week and use the tube to commute. You are struggling to get into work because of your symptoms. You live with your boyfriend who is supportive. You do not smoke or drink.
ICE: You are finding the commute unbearable and don't know what to do. You think you may lose your job if you tell your boss what's happening. You are also concerned there is something wrong with your heart.

Instructions for the examiner:

Elicits the presenting complaint (1)
Asks the following—chest tightness, palpitations, tingling, link to using the tube, history of anxiety (5)
Asks about past medical history, and family history (2)
Asks about social history (1)
asks about ICE (1)
Total (10)

This patient is struggling with panic attacks triggered by using the tube. She may benefit from treatment with propranolol or an SSRI.

I hope you found this book useful. It has been designed as a guide to help you identify what disease to exclude when taking a history. You will have to read around the topics. I would recommend photocopying or recreating the tables to use during your revision.

The most important thing to improve history taking skills is to practise, practice practice!

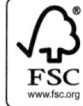

MIX
Papier aus verantwortungsvollen Quellen
Paper from responsible sources
FSC® C105338

If you have any concerns about our products,
you can contact us on
ProductSafety@springernature.com

In case Publisher is established outside the EU,
the EU authorized representative is:
**Springer Nature Customer Service Center GmbH
Europaplatz 3, 69115 Heidelberg, Germany**

Printed by Libri Plureos GmbH
in Hamburg, Germany